# The Buddha in Our Bellies

Keith Robinson with Yoshiko Robinson

Sensitivity Warning:

*The Buddha in Our Bellies* tells stories of transforming suffering from Crohn's disease and identity issues into fulfillment, joy, and fellowship. Both the suffering and the transformation have been messy. As such, a few descriptions of bowel movements and medical procedures are told. Readers might find these disturbing. *The Buddha in Our Bellies* also contains indirect, not graphic, references to domestic violence, sexual violence, and military atrocities. For privacy reasons, some names, dates, and locations have been changed.

Copyright © 2023 by Keith Robinson and Yoshiko Robinson
All Rights Reserved. No part of this publication may be reproduced, stored in a retrieval system, or transmitted, in any form or in any means — by electronic, mechanical, photocopying, recording or otherwise — without prior written permission, except as permitted by the laws of Canada.
For permissions, write pilgrimsofjoy@gmail.com

ISBN(s)
978-1-7389115-0-9 (print)
978-93-93262-33-2 (India)
9798391982159 (KDP)
B0C2RTN8LM (Asin)

Drawings by Yoshiko Robinson, other than Vesalius print and map.
Original brushwork figure by Keith Robinson.
Design by Shida Studio Inc. <https://shidastudio.com>
Photo of authors by Thibeau Nonier, Toulon.
Back cover gouache watercolour, *winter walk,* by Chiu Lin Wong.
Map of India by Black Pearl Film Works.

The primary text font is EB Garamond, a modern open source implementation of the classic mid-sixteenth century typefaces of the Parisian engraver and punch-cutter Claude Garamont. EB Garamond is licensed by SIL Open Font License (OFL).
<https://scripts.sil.org/cms/scripts/page.php?site_id=nrsi&id=OFL>

Special Elite font, used for Out There chapter and Sister Carmelita letter, mimics Smith Corona Special Elite type NR6. Apache 2.0 license for print, digital, and commercial use.
<https://www.fontsquirrel.com/license/special-elite>

To our mentor, Daisaku Ikeda.

And to the thousands of dedicated people worldwide who devote every waking moment to relieving the misery of Crohn's disease.

# CONTENTS

| | |
|---|---|
| PREFACE | IX |
| INTRODUCTION | XII |
| AUTHORS' NOTES | XVI |
| EPIGRAPH | XVII |
| PROLOGUE | XVIII |
| PART ONE | 1 |
| ORIGINS | |
| I am a pilgrim | 2 |
| Taken Out of Paradise | 5 |
| A Green Room | 8 |
| We Are the Shadow People | 11 |
| My Stomach Hurt | 15 |
| Not a New Disease | 21 |
| The Festival | 29 |
| "No team wants you." | 34 |
| The Swan | 39 |
| This Is Real | 43 |
| Inflamed, Invisible | 47 |
| The Asura, Inflammation Personified | 54 |

| | |
|---|---|
| Part of the World | 59 |
| "For those who work for peace." | 64 |
| In the Middle of Something | 71 |
| "I trust you, Yo-chan." | 73 |
| PART TWO  
DEPARTURES | 90 |
| The Thinnest Hope | 91 |
| Siddhartha's Departure | 97 |
| Students and Teachers | 104 |
| Out There | 109 |
| Siddhartha's Quest | 119 |
| My Quest | 129 |
| Courage | 151 |
| Siddhartha's Fall | 152 |
| My Fall | 154 |
| "Yo-chan, we will meet again." | 161 |
| after-death in three verses | 171 |
| "Ask for Yoshiko." | 172 |
| I Will Never Forget His Eyes. | 178 |
| The Striving | 187 |
| The Awakening | 197 |
| PART THREE  
AWAKENINGS | 207 |
| wait with me | 208 |
| Mom and Dad | 210 |

| | |
|---|---|
| The Hungry Ghost | 218 |
| Lean Forward | 234 |
| Stephen's Story | 236 |
| Coming Home | 249 |
| Gut Feelings | 253 |
| "Yoshiko, do something. Please." | 261 |
| The Buddha's Friend | 268 |
| Friday the 13th | 277 |
| Belonging | 287 |
| The Ferry | 290 |
| The Maestro | 292 |
| Gardening in the Loire | 297 |
| Blue Buddhas Make Me Whole | 300 |
| New Year's Morning, 2021 | 311 |
| The Hill | 313 |
| The question of the bench | 318 |
| EPILOGUE | 320 |
| MY GLOSSARY | 323 |
| ACKNOWLEDGEMENTS | 326 |
| 1. RESOURCES | 328 |
| Endnotes | 329 |

# PREFACE

"Crohn's disease — isn't that where you poop and poop and then you die?" — a ten-year-old

"People like you often get Crohn's." — a doctor

"I wish I had Crohn's disease to lose weight." — a bulimic friend

"Just remove gluten from your diet. You will be cured almost immediately." — a colleague

"It's all in your head." — more people than I can remember

"You eat too fast." — Dad

In 1968, after years of illness, I received a diagnosis of regional enteritis, now called Crohn's disease (CD). With Crohn's, the body's immune system treats its digestive tract as a foreign object.

Not a death sentence, the diagnosis became a life-sentence. Nothing could be done. The pain and exhaustion I endured daily would continue or worsen. The disease might destroy any part of my digestive tract, from mouth to anus. My body harboured a hidden rebellion against my guts, inflaming, twisting and ripping holes in them. My future was to suffer unseen as a drained, pain-stricken freak. How would I get through a semester, let alone a lifetime? No girl will want me. The prognosis was for endless surgeries, my guts replaced by a bag, dying of malnutrition, or a long, lonely torment, pooping myself to death.

What had I done to deserve this? I wished it went away. I hated my guts and myself. For decades following the diagnosis, I believed my situation remained not just unique but uniquely unique. That no words existed to describe my life with Crohn's. That no one cares about my bowel movements, and certainly no one wants to read a book about them.

Fatigue from Crohn's and other autoimmune diseases differs from normal fatigue caused by insufficient sleep or over-exertion. According to *Harvard Health Publishing*, "For many people with autoimmune disease, fatigue is the most debilitating symptom.... It's a feeling of constant exhaustion that makes it hard to get through the day, let alone participate in activities...."[1] Writer and poet Meghan O'Rourke describes her own: "... autoimmune fatigue is different from a sleep-deprived person's exhaustion. The worst part of my fatigue, the one I couldn't explain to anyone — I knew I'd seem crazy — was the loss of an intact sense of self."[2]

Autoimmune disease and CD can destroy our connection to who we are. *The Buddha in Our Bellies* is concerned with my transformation of both the "loss of an intact sense of self" and the physical experience of CD.

An immune system disorder behaves something like organ transplant rejection. In addition to the physical symptoms of Crohn's, I experienced a kind of psychic rejection. We will see how the guts form the physical basis of non-physical qualities — courage, will, and foundational sense of identity. I also rejected my guts' intuition and imagination.

I can not change the fact I have a chronic, life-long, often debilitating disease. But my response to my sickness defines my experience. I didn't choose Crohn's. I chose my response. My future of pain, fatigue, and loneliness has become a present of joy and purpose, even a calling. And now I know: I'm not alone.

## Let me set the table

As a kid, even if my stomach hurt, I set the table for dinner. That was my task, and I enjoyed it. It wasn't all fancy, and I didn't turn cloth napkins into roses, but I figured out how many forks on the left and whether we needed steak knives. We had a massive oak dining table with leaves. If guests were coming, I had to figure out how many leaves and, little me, open the table, carry the heavy leaves, and put them in place.

Often the family dinners themselves ended in family fights, but that's not my fault. I just set the table. When people came over, I had to be extra attentive to what bowls and cutlery to put out and whether to polish the fancy silver. Spreading out newspaper to contain the mess, I used a rag and a tin can of Twinkle Silver Polish. My fingers worked the creamy polish into the crevices and curves of the old Hungarian cutlery.

Later in life, I cooked dinners for family and friends and clients and set lots of tables. I enjoy it. Once dinner starts, I don't have to talk or be the centre of attention. Just set the table and people will figure out the rest. Let the conversation and the good times flow.

I became a sommelier. A sommelier brings the efforts of a sincere, hard-working winegrower and a sincere, hard-working chef to a sincere guest. We find a bottle that matches the three to the occasion and the season and company. We open it and pour it and get out of the way. Those times we get it right, the guest experiences bliss; we make memories. Lives change.

I became a manager and host of short-term rental properties. Travellers belong, feel at home, in the spaces Yoshiko and I create. They can enjoy a memorable life experience in a strange city, even for a few nights. The romantic getaway on the surface may be a last shot for a couple in crisis. A typical business trip might be a career on the brink. A family vacation might be the summer of a lifetime. All the pilgrimages of life.

Over time, I learned these skills. Respect the guest; anticipate their needs. Prepare every detail. Generosity. Latitude. Set the table. Pull the cork. Get out of the way.

As I learned to make room for others, I learned to make room for my own disowned character. Possibility and imagination have found space in my life. Hopefully, some of these skills arrive at the pages of this book. I set the table for you, dear reader. Set out these tales of hardship and uncertainty and possibility. Have a seat.

# INTRODUCTION

*In my Book of Memory in the early part
where there is little to be read,
there comes a chapter with the rubric:
Incipit vita nova [The new life begins].*
Dante Alighieri[3]

WE LIVE IN PERILOUS times. Climate change and nuclear destruction threaten every one of us. No pope or president, guru or general, is going to save us. One way or another, we will have to save ourselves, live together, and share our beautiful Earth. The only solution I offer is connection. I wrote *The Buddha in Our Bellies* hoping to connect with one other suffering, caring person. May my story of finding hope in misery connect to yours.

The Buddha in my belly knows we ride this boat of life on planet Earth together; we sink, swim, or get to the other side together. My perspective is that of engagement with the here and now. I tried running away. It didn't work.

Whether by nature, nurture, God's will, karma, chance or choice, here we are. Rich, poor, healthy, sick, fearful, or foolhardy, this is us. We can't escape reality; we may as well face it. We just might change it.

*The Buddha in Our Bellies* weaves memory, history, imagination, dream, mythology, and poetry. It shows how two people dealt with their reality and struggled to move forward with kindness, creativity, and purpose.

I was a middle-class Jewish-Canadian kid with an incurable disease. Unable to change my family or my illness, I sought a way to change myself.

Yoshiko grew up in an isolated village on the side of a mountain in Japan. Her father survived Soviet forced labour camps and her mother, a post-war refugee, walked across northern Asia. Although Yoshiko's childhood was far from carefree, she was wild and happy. She longed to see the wider world, nurturing a dream to contribute to peace and harmony. Yoshiko wrote her stories and drew the book's illustrations, except where noted. With her help, I wrote the rest.

A third character whose stories I tell died twenty-five centuries ago. Siddhartha was the scion of an ancient Indian agrarian clan. From his childhood on, questions of identity and purpose tormented him. All beings seemed destined to suffer in life and die without meaning. He became the Buddha, the Enlightened One. In his angst, courage, and resolution, I find inspiration and parallels. I also speculate about his relationship with three remarkable women: the wife he abandoned, who became a ferocious disciple and equal; the milkmaid who saved him; and a grief-stricken soul who became his friend.

I do not intend my tales of the Buddha's life as a definitive history or biography. They are no more valid than any other recounting of the life of this amazing man. My accounts reflect my research, biases, experiences, expectations, doubts, and hopes.

*The Buddha in Our Bellies* will travel to forests of ancient India, witness a seventeenth century autopsy in a Swiss morgue, seek an unknown father in a cemetery in Queens, New York; get lost, sick, and hungry in Paris; meet outlaws, farmers, arrogant priests, a giant looking for a mate and a mission, the lonely, the forgotten, and the enlightened.

Since I am neither a medical practitioner nor a Buddhist scholar, my authority is only of my experience and studies. I am a spokesperson only of my opinions.

This book won't tell you how to change your life, how to cure Crohn's, or how to practise Buddhism. It will tell how our lives grew and of our growing belief that all people can change theirs.

The message of these stories: break free of limitations to become the person we believe ourselves to be. Here and there you will find my amateur poetry to convey my heart and guts, in places where the head is inadequate. I hope you enjoy them.

My life has been a quest, embarked on with unsteady steps. At first I longed for relief from pain; I wanted to be like others. In time, my quest took me in unexpected directions, to transform my self-disgust into empathy and fellowship. My path of restoration and healing began in an odd place: my broken belly. From my belly — charred, carved, and scarred — came the qualities of the Buddha, the highest self, my liberation. I write from my gut to you, from my most sacred intuition to yours.

The idea of a Buddha in one's belly, of course, is metaphor, referring to our highest qualities being inherent within us already. Beyond metaphor, research is finding that the gut is the source of inspiration, courage, and core sense of identity.

---

Neurogastroenterology is the study of our gut's influence on our mood, health, and thoughts. Our digestive system, pancreas, and gallbladder hold our enteric brain. Food passing through the gut is still external to us. Only after digestion does it become internal, part of us. With roughly half as many neurons as the big brain, the gut constantly communicates with the brain and other organs. The gut sends messages slowly by releasing hormones, quickly through glutamate, and almost instantly by triggering the vagus nerve with serotonin.

The gut microbiome is bigger than the brain. Trillions of bacteria, fungi, parasites, and viruses in our gut total about 2 kilograms. The brain in our skull weighs about 1.4 kilograms. Research is finding how our microbiome affects our mental and physical health. Our gut health influences everything from depression to cancers.

The brain symbolizes the centre of our intellect; the heart, the source of emotion; and the gut, our intuition. The word guts means strength (a gutsy move) and intuition (gut feeling, a gut check). Research is learning these symbolic meanings have their basis in biology. As my guts found acceptance in my body, and as I found belonging in the world, I learned to welcome the intuitive, the imagined and wondrous.

And the Buddha? Who or what is that? The Buddha is not a supernatural being; neither god nor deity. Rather, Buddha was a real person who lived in India around the fifth century BCE. He gained the very human qualities of wisdom, compassion, and life-force. He believed everyone equally could access these qualities. Scattered through this book are stories of his life, his fears, longings, and hopes.

My unhealthy gut became my motivation to change and grow. From my guts, the source of so much pain and misery, emerged those same Buddha-like qualities of insight, empathy, and life-force.

Yoshiko and I practise Buddhism with Soka Gakkai (The Value Creation Society), a modern world-wide movement for peace, education, and culture. How we each came to practise with Soka Gakkai is told herein.

Buddhism and medicine, like most subjects, have their share of specialized language. I've tried to keep the insider language out. My intention was to use a minimum of jargon. A short GLOSSARY at the end defines my usage of terms. Also, at the book's end, a RESOURCES page offers sources of additional information on Crohn's disease (CD), hidradenitis suppurativa (HS), and Soka Buddhism.

# AUTHORS' NOTES

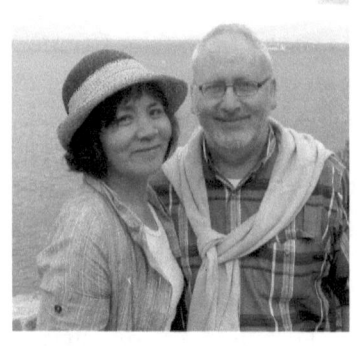

THIS IS A WORK of memory, history, and imagination, and is subject to the strengths and weaknesses of each. We've combined people into one character, and omitted many important people. Likely, others' memories of these events are more accurate. We've gone to significant efforts to ensure the accuracy of the history. Any errors are our own. We hope the stories of imagination are the truest of them all.

The genre of memoir is growing like a wild vine in exciting directions and subgenres — lyric, collage, speculative. *The Buddha in Our Bellies* contains elements of speculative memoir, making space for the imagined and the wondrous. Outer events in our lives link to hidden inner realms. The Chilean writer Isabel Allende said, "A memoir is my version of events. My perspective. I choose what to tell and what to omit. I choose the adjectives to describe a situation, and in that sense, I'm creating a form of fiction."[4]

All memoir springs from subjective memory, out of the unique perspective and interpretation of the narrator. We wish to share the meaning, not the events, of our experience. For in that meaning we connect with you.

With love and appreciation to you for reading these tales, from the Buddhas in our bellies, Keith and Yoshiko.

*A great human revolution in just a single individual will help achieve a change in the destiny of a nation and further, will enable a change in the destiny of all humankind.*[5]
Daisaku Ikeda

# PROLOGUE

> The prayer bells are ringing
> hurry, hurry, hurry
> Leaves are falling,
> the sun is setting
> hurry, hurry, hurry
>
> Storms are gathering,
> Your hair is on fire
> Your temples are burning
> Mice are scurrying
> hurry, hurry, hurry
>
> Life is fleeting,
> death is waiting
> hurry, hurry, hurry
>
> Time is a pyre
> hurry, hurry, hurry.

## Government Office, Los Angeles, 1975

AFTER WAITING WEEKS FOR an appointment, I trudged in desperate and unprepared and out of options.

Bare office. Three metal desks, two unoccupied. At one, I watched an angular black woman with graying hair working, with a telephone, a binder holding forms, and a couple of mismatched pens. Her desktop lay as barren as her flat expression: no notepads or in/out trays, no stationery holder, no lamp, no cup for stale coffee. No flower vase warmed the space, no photo frame, nothing personal.

Cold, functional space. I waited across the desk, in a hard metal chair, clueless how this worked, trying to get a read on her. For my sake, I hoped that eight hours a day in this humourless office didn't freeze her every drop of care and kindness. For her sake, too.

Two framed pictures hung on the wall: Jerry Brown and Gerald Ford. Two Jerries running things; that's kind of funny. Crack a joke. Her dismal eyes said she needed a laugh. My joking mouth opened, then shut. Another frame hung on the wall behind her, a certificate or diploma.

She opened the binder, grasped a pen. Those bony fingers held my fate. "Tell me your situation, Mr. uh, Robinson?"

I'd stuffed rent receipts, bills, an eviction notice, in my pocket. They stayed stuffed.

"Yeah. All right, so, I've got no money, no food, no job. I can't make rent. Nowhere to go if I'm booted out. I won't even have a car to sleep in. They repossessed my car in the middle of the night. I hid the Pinto and pulled off the distributor rotor to disable the car, but they found it, towing it out from the bushes."

There it is, lady, that's me. Most of it, anyway. That's how I got here, towed out from under bushes. Now you got almost everything.

She scribbled a note. "But you can work?"

Work. Stealing car stereos and selling them. Stealing from John, Stan and Kathy. This wasn't work. My pathetic attempt to obtain welfare crumbled before it began.

"Mr. Robinson?"

"I have Crohn's disease."

"What's that? A disability?"

"It's a disease." Tell her about the hospital. It wouldn't matter. She doesn't care about surgery. No, simply tell her.

"Are you sick now?"

Bile rose in my mouth; a cramp began.

Speak. Don't sabotage this. I'm sick. I need this; open your stupid mouth, you putz, and tell her. Not strong enough to survive on the streets, I'll be dead in short order.

This place is not for me. Welfare exists for poor people, the girlfriends and wives of the guys inside. But I need to eat. Please, I don't deserve this. I don't deserve welfare. Show her. Show her my belly. Lift my shirt so she sees inside, the sutures coming out oozing. She'll see the hole leaking puss, the hole large enough for her scrawny ice-shard fingers. Allow her to see my belly wriggle exposed and punctured, like a bloated, greasy fish on a hook.

"Sort of. I guess not. I got out of jail a couple of weeks ago."

"For what, Mr. Robinson?" She leans back. Head tilted, eyes doubtful.

"Nothing much. Scofflaw." My face tingled, hot. Bit my cheeks. Harder. That's all this meant: a form to be filed, a file to be closed.

"There aren't any programs for you." She scanned me, a fish slice on display, a bastard bug in a jar. Then she put down the pen. "You are employable. Any friends who can be of assistance? Family?"

Been stealing money from my friends. That's them assisting.

"My parents are in Canada." The cramps spread from my guts to my thighs, then all the way to the base of my skull. Twisting in my chair. Nothing new about the cramps, but nothing I got used to. Trouble hearing what she said, but it must be some version of no. Gotta get out of here, clear out.

"Canada?" She's closing the binder. "You don't qualify for Social Assistance. You are employable. Find a job."

I found a toilet in the nick of time.

# PART ONE
# ORIGINS

In the crucible
flames, pressure, exertion
preparing the void

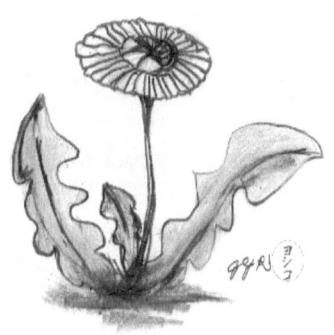

# I am a pilgrim

I am a pilgrim,
wandering in lands strange and fair
Treading a new path
Treading paths well paved
Searching for them holy sites,
the sacred, the unnamed,
and the profane,
Searching for the whole and ripe.
Like a snail, slowly,
with home on my back
Searching for the broken,
the forgotten, the insane.

Once I was not a pilgrim,
those tired days I scoured every side road.
Is that my way home?
Craning my neck to see 'round every bend.
Wondering is home just past there?
Back there?
Knocking on doors,
"I think I may have come from here.
Mind if I look around?"
Wondering where . . . where was mine?

# I AM A PILGRIM

The folks I met,
some helpful, some not
— princes and priests and paupers —
None knew my land,
none knew my way back.
Many had advice for my way forward
—Take this supplement, read this book,
let's get coffee, how yah doin'?

I met animals too,
but not very well.
Animals frightened me
— what they knew, their posture
Back then I was not a pilgrim,
but alone, aimless, homeless

One day I met a snail
— small, like me; slow, like me.
I quizzed the snail,
"do you know the way home?"
The snail did not understand,
for it carried its home everywhere.
Ever forward, never running,
carefully.

So, I became a pilgrim,
from fields away.
Treading a one-way path
— forward but with twists and turns
and long delays,
Searching for them holy sites,
new-built or relic
Searching for the whole and torn,
Like a snail, slowly,
building home for others,
Sometimes lost, forgotten, delayed.

Now I'm a pilgrim
from a foreign land
I seek the outcasts,
venoms and their elixirs,
the vine, all beauty.
Rumi's ecstasy.
I seek microbes,
connections divine and bitter.

I'm a pilgrim of no tribe.
All my energy goes to roam this earth
Given wholly to wander this garden,
this desert, this brook.
Now older, perhaps I won't shirk
from the animals,
perhaps take a horse as a teacher.

# Taken Out of Paradise

## Announcement, Kerrisdale, Vancouver, 1961

IN HIS MEMOIRS, *An Urban Life Journey*, my father described his Vancouver days as "teaching in paradise." He pulled us out of paradise for a job at a consulting firm in San Francisco.

Dad gathered us in the living room of our Kerrisdale home for his announcement. He stood, pipe in one hand, scotch in the other, head tilted back. We parked ourselves to listen, Stevie and me on the couch, Peter on the piano stool, Mom and Rags on the floor, his curly red head in her lap. Dad faced us, his back to the picture window over West 34 Ave. Through the window, the spring afternoon rains paused. Our neighbour, Mrs. Campbell, gardened. Dad spoke a bit too loud. "The students and faculty at UBC have been wonderful, but I'm eager to return to the States. A major research and policy study in San Francisco recruited me personally to head it."

Moving to California. Going somewhere different. Exciting. Stevie and Peter appeared serious, not excited, figuring out what this meant. Mom took a drag on her cigarette, leaned towards the ashtray half-hidden by Rag's paw.

Too excited to stay still, I whizzed out to the front porch and yelled, "Mrs. Campbell, I have news. We're moving to the United States. Dad's recruited personally." A hand on my shoulder directed me inside the house. Dad's smile evaporated, replaced by his more usual disappointed face. I did the wrong thing. I was wrong. We don't announce we are moving.

So, I fetched a suitcase from a closet to pack and began stuffing it with a lamp, my sneakers. What else can I cram in? My brothers, still sitting, glanced at each other. What a kid. Wrong again. Moving a family took more than a suitcase; moving means a big deal, bigger than a suitcase.

## The Bogeyman

Over the following days, moving kept Mom busy. She packed and organized and figured out what to do with Rags. Paperwork swamped Mom because Stephen and I weren't Americans, and leaving us in Vancouver "wasn't practical." She needed to sell the house. Strangers talked about buying and selling my home, while wandering through the piles of papers and boxes. And she phoned the school every day for Peter's records since he skipped two grades. She had to arrange for schools in California to accept him so young and for his piano lessons. And what to tell us about Rags, about Dad flying back and forth to San Francisco and buying a house? Giant, important preparations.

Mom rarely mentioned the bogeyman, the bogeyman from the old country. When she did, leaning above us, she meant it. Or she seemed to mean it. With people coming through and me at her feet trying to help, she'd say, "Ol' Keith, if I trip over you another time, the bogeyman will come to get you." I didn't see any bogeymen. She couldn't be serious. But what if it came at night, in dark clothes and dark glasses and their enormous hats cloaking their mean face? Their mule pulled their dark cart with a cage and chains and a huge lock. Mom knew things, and Gramma, the daughter of a Hungarian princess, knew people from back in Europe. Mom sure sounded serious. Find somewhere to help, but not with the important things.

When Dad came back home, they fought. They fought about us three, the house. "You bought a house before we received an offer here? In San Francisco without my seeing it? How could you do that?" Both raised their voices, hardness in their tone.

Mom came from San Francisco. She loved San Francisco for its open-minded, progressive culture. But preparing to return home didn't make her happy. Maybe San Francisco wasn't so neat. She said, "I am going to lie down for a few minutes, good ol' Keith. The boils." Her face said both kill and cry.

I didn't want her crying or killing me. Where to go, what should I do? San Francisco started sounding less exciting than before, but I couldn't stay home. I tried being a grownup and leaving, but barely got as far as the corner house. They sent Rags to drag the escapee back, and besides, running away scared me. And I tried being a kid and crying but my brothers made fun of me.

Since Mom went to bed, I read *Yertle the Turtle* in Stevie and my room. I adored Mack, the smallest turtle; he stood up to the dictator Yertle. Mean Yertle didn't scare Mack. Or, even scared, Mack didn't care. He overthrew the dictator and freed the other turtles.

Also, Mom needed to finish editing and typing Dad's dissertation. And, she said, she researched and wrote it. Farewell events and choosing a cover for his book kept Dad busy, too. He planned to take us for a clubhouse sandwich at the faculty club to bid farewell to the staff. But I came down with a fever and Stevie didn't want to go and Pete had a piano lesson.

I didn't understand research or dissertations. If I wasn't sick, if I grew up, I could help, make Mom happy. But I was sick. My fever made me dozy, white sores in my mouth, and cough kept me half awake. I tried to stay awake, in case the bogeyman proved real and came after me. I pressed my loose tooth with my tongue. It hurt a good hurt and kept me awake, so I did that. I lay in bed with thoughts of being taken and something Dad said. Dad, being Navy, explained that on board they labelled items to be stowed until arrival, "not wanted on voyage." That fit me.

# A Green Room

## San Francisco, September 3, 1961

THE TEMPERATURE REACHED 92 °F, about 20 degrees above normal for early September. Mom arranged for me to start grade two at Alamo Elementary School on the 5th. I wouldn't make it. I was sick with measles and quarantined for a few days at US Immigration. Everybody continued on ahead to set up our home.

I wake up. It's hot. My head is hot. The air is hot and heavy, pressing me down. Pressing me into a green bed. This isn't my bed. Where am I? Green everywhere. My clothes are green, a green robe. Under the robe, my chest has red spots. My arms too. I resemble a pizza in a spinach box. The walls are green. The walls are moving. I hear voices speaking, too fast for me to follow. A typewriter goes clickety-clack. Where am I? Is this death?

Not dead, I am sick. Lying on a green cot, surrounded by green curtains. Waiting for my family to come get me. Waiting to get better. Too hot to do anything and nowhere to go. The people here won't allow me to go anywhere. The Americans. They declared me contagious. I'm catchable.

Nothing to do. Wait. Everybody's gone to the new house. I open T*he Cat in the Hat* on the cot with green sheets, but it's too hot to read. I try my *Book of Haiku,* but the words don't make sense. At least the cough isn't as bad. The P.A. hums and howls so loud I can't read.

The curtain moves. Somebody's there. Please don't hurt me. I wish they'd talk to me, tell me what is going on, or take me out of here. Maybe I dreamt that someone came. My head's hot. Floaty. Dreamy. Did they slip in to fetch me and leave 'cause I was sleeping? Will someone take me home?

Americans speak fast. They speak too fast, over the P.A. Everything takes so long, so slow.

Today, Teddy tried to escape again. Poor Teddy, with his smashed nose and missing eye from leaping out of the car. There, under the cot; he must have climbed down. I couldn't reach him and now he's gone. Come back, please, Teddy. I hope they return to take me to the new place, but Teddy has to come back first.

The lights are always on. Day and night. I can tell it's evening by the food tray left inside the curtain. The paper on the tray reads "Dinner meal, minor." At night, they pull up the sides of the cot. Outside, not as noisy, not as many voices speaking fast, less clickety-clack.

They say I am sick. What if I'm dying? If I die, I'd better prepare. Figure out death, what happens after I die. Going up to heaven or down to hell makes no sense. I am here. My body is here. What's the idea? Someone turns up with a long black station wagon and drives me down or up? That's too silly. C'mon. Don't be stupid. Sure, figure it out. Find my drawing pad. Open eyes.

A small table next to my cot holds my stuff: books, my Pacific Industrial Polar Bear toothbrush in a cup, and Teddy when he's not in bed or running away.

Pete said I must be careful not to lose my toothbrush, that "America doesn't benefit from Pacific Industrial Polar Bear toothbrushes." I am glad to be from a country with clean teeth and people who speak slow enough so I can follow.

All right, grab my drawing pad and pencil from the table. Let's see. Draw a line and me underneath, lying dead. This line shows the ground. Dirt. Here's me, buried under. Dead. Above the ground, people parading back and forth across the paper. Not dead. Draw them. Stick people, they don't look real. That's okay. As long as they're not dead, no one cares how they look.

I can draw lines from my body to them. I can be any of them. That might be how death goes. Or close to that. Squeeze shut my eyes and think about this, figure out death. If I die here, I need to know.

I wake up. There's movement in the corner of the green room. A mountain lion on a cliff, about to leap. ready to leap over the bed's metal sides and pounce on me. Don't rip me. Scream. I am going to die. No, don't make any noise. Stay quiet. It might leave.

I wake up again. Teddy lies back on the table. He climbed back up when I slept. Please don't run away again. No mountain lion. No cliff. A stack of green robes and towels lie on a steel cabinet in the corner. It's a trick. The towels' fold formed the lion's back. The knobs on the drawer, its eyes. I see. So when I go to sleep next, I should face away from that corner so I don't wake up to the scary mountain lion again. Sure, but when I sleep I roll over. Maybe I should go to sleep facing the corner, then when I turn over and wake up I won't spot it.

Safest not to sleep. Sure. That will work.

A radio blares lots of talk and some music. They talk too fast, but I catch a little, about a heat wave. Hey, that's the song, "What'd I say?" Pete taught me to play the left hand on the piano and he'd play all over with both hands.

If Petey was here, he'd figure out what to say. He'd talk to the people, the Americans, tell them to take care of his little brother. Or Stevie. Stevie would play with me. Make me laugh. Steve and Pete left too, needed to do the important stuff. It's too hot and everybody's gone besides Teddy. Only broken Teddy and the green pillow.

# We Are the Shadow People

WHILE RESEARCHING THIS BOOK, I read an article in *Tricycle Magazine* that mentioned obscure hells inhabited by forgotten, miserable souls.[6] These hells, called *lokāntarikā* in Buddhist mythology, exist in-between normal space, in complete darkness. The *lokāntarikā* are totally isolated; their inhabitants alone and abandoned. The plight of the trapped beings startled me, touched me. I felt their story inside, not on the magazine page. The mention was brief, an aside; the article's focus lay elsewhere.

I've dubbed the suffering beings who dwell in these between-spaces hells, "shadow people." Akin to the shadow people, I suffered unseen. "Please witness us, hidden and tormented. Hear our silenced cries." Like them, I found a spark of hope.

Buddhist scriptures describe a vast array of hells and, in excruciating detail, the torments the condemned suffer. They are not eternally damned, despite extraordinarily lengthy sentences, often measured in aeons. Burning hells exist, as well as frozen hells and subsidiary hells and a hell of incessant suffering. There are feces hells and sharp thorn hells and a blood red lotus hell. Each hell neatly matches the damned's evil causes.

Obscurity veils the lokāntarikā hell. The canon defines these between-spaces hells as dark and isolated spaces where light can not reach. The inhabitants of these hells believe themselves alone.

The in-between spaces exist where cosmic orbs (something like solar systems) meet. Inside the orbs, suns shine light. Outside, in-between the orbs is only a dark void. Consider three coins or three marbles, converging edge to edge. Where they touch forms the curved sides of a tetrahedral-like space, outside the margins of any universe. These benighted spaces form the unlit cells holding this hell's denizens. The walls press against the inmates, immobilising them, pinning their legs. They can't move to escape. The cell that is the shadow people's entire world seals tight, without exits. No way out. No light in.

The stories tell nothing of the wretched inmates of these horrid crypts; or what evil causes they committed. We aren't told how to avoid their fate ourselves. That's how obscure these hells are, how forgotten are the shadow people. It seems their very existence caused their banishment. Punished for being who they are, neither divine judgement nor their own poor choices condemned them.

The shadow people dwell in the supernatural, mythic realm of scripture, yes. We uncover them here on Earth as well, in alleys, basements, refugee camps, and locked away, forgotten in long-term care. They live in the cracks in-between, often drugged, their bodies emptied, their minds stolen, or their sex bought and sold.

Utter darkness shrouds the inhabitants. They cannot see themselves. They can't sense their own arms, their gift to embrace and build. Unable to sense themselves, they lose inspiration, creativity, and their sense of wonder. Darkness cloaks their highest selves — their nobility, courage, and resilience.

## An in-between space hell

Once upon a time, in an unlit, airless in-between space, knelt a lone naked figure. Male, although plenty of shadow people are not male. The bowed walls pinched this shadow person in a vise, pressing. He knelt in submission, with no clothes, belongings, or any token of identity. His head and torso squeezed into a ball, curled as a dung beetle rolled in terror. His lungs frozen, neither expanding nor contracting. No wind carried screams or whimpers. Lightless, airless. Breathless, he did not die.

The dungeon's walls bowed his body, obscuring his face but exposing his genitals. What demons or warders rule this nightmare prison stay hidden.

Others drift past, unseen, darker than shadow. With no air to carry sound, they passed unheard. Like phantoms from different dimensions, they glide through the same space, concealed from each other. Drifting past each other, in isolation, each certain of their solitude.

The darkness crushed both day and night. Unable to sleep, he descended into a waking nightmare. He forgot how long he'd been there, whether one minute or one minute less than eternity. Neither pulse nor heartbeat measured time. He forgot any earlier life. His own name: he forgot his name and who he'd been.

Yet he remained conscious, or semi-conscious. Shards of images punctured his mind, as if poisoned or hallucinating. He dreamt the dreams of the sedated. And in the dreams he confused wakefulness with sleep. His deserted nightmare held neither friends nor enemies, void of dream monsters or demons. Not even nightmare spirits slipped in or out of sleep. He dreamt forsaken and sleepless. Hopeless in the unbreaking dawn. Sleepless in a waking nightmare.

Blood didn't pulse in his throat. His guts didn't growl, no acrid taste on his palate. The crypt walls pinched against his curved back. Wall scraping bone. Back contorting his neck, buckling his head, face drooping into chest; ribs squeezed into the lungs, into his yielding knees. The cell moulded him into its form, shaping him, expunging whoever he'd been.

Pinched and bent in darkness, he lost his identity by being himself. He is invisible and unacceptable on account of who he is — of colour or disabled or indigenous or sick or gender non-binary or simply different. He slipped into the in-between spaces. It's easy to collapse, when invisible. When no one sees, no one cares.

## A light within

> *The dark and secluded places within those in-between lands, where the light of the sun and the moon can never penetrate, were all brightly illuminated and the living beings were all able to see one another, and they all exclaimed, saying, 'How is it that living beings have suddenly come into existence in this place?'*[57]
> The Lotus Sutra

The man remained in darkness. But, beyond his tortured mind's awareness, beyond interoception, something stirred. In the darkest recesses of his entrails, in the shade inside shade, a spark refused to be extinguished. Light reached his eyes. Painful light. He squeezed his lids against the pain. He detected a beat. A beat, known, yet forgotten. Holding the breath, please, please, please. And a gasp.

Breath came in tiny, shallow, unfamiliar bursts. The light brought air. Breath. Limbs tingled. With each breath, more air. Air filling his lungs, streaming in his arteries. Air expanded into his in-between cell. The space inflated, flooded with light and air. The moment held dread and frail hope.

He opened one eye a sliver, then the other. Blinked. The beetle uncurled, his back straightening, one painful vertebra by one.

Here are arms, hands. Tears. Somebody abides there. Here. Not alone.

The light originated not from outside, but from a hidden inner lamp. Others emerged. He recognized brethren and sistren, discovered himself among them. And look, a shadow, his shadow from his light. The first light glows, self-lit.

The eyes open not to the sun-kissed blossoms nor the moon-lit tides, not the arms, nor the lungs, but to others. His arms widened to the others. Stretch, jump. The others stretch and leap, mouths agape, sparkling into beams, bursting with joy at recognizing others.

These are the abandoned shadow people, the outcasts, outlaws, and freaks. Their light illuminates the darkest hells.

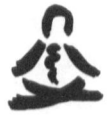

# My Stomach Hurt

## The smartest eight-year-old, San Francisco, 1962

FOR MUCH OF CHILDHOOD, this or that infection moved through me. After the measles, a fever-ridden staph infection laid me low. The staph caused rashes on my face and arms with pus-filled blisters. After recovering from staph, I suffered bouts of strep throat, followed by more staph. Somewhere in the back and forth, stomach cramps began, then diarrhea and fatigue.

In the schoolyard at Alamo Elementary, I cornered the brainiest eight-year-old. "You know how when you first wake up, you are still tired until you get going? Then, at bedtime, you tire again, then it's time to go to sleep? What happens when the first tired grows longer and longer and the second tired gets longer and there's no time I'm not tired? No matter how much I sleep?"

Suzie Wong tilted her head, adjusting imaginary glasses to inspect me, a three headed bastard bug in a jar. "See a doctor. You're dying."

At home, Dad said, "You aren't dying. You eat too fast." The doctor said my pain originated in my head. Mom, when not bedridden herself, took me to other doctors. The other doctors tested with vague results. No one treated my head.

## The tunnel, Early 1960s

We moved twice in San Francisco, both times in the west end, Richmond District. We stayed within a quick bike ride to the sprawling military base, the Presidio, or the rectangular park that bisects the city, Golden Gate Park. Both the Presidio and the park enjoyed plenty of natural areas with places to hide. Through the gaps in the fences, among the woods and undergrowth, I hid my three-speed and climbed into my private green nest.

Twice I began excavating a tunnel with a shovel in our backyard for a below-ground hideout. But Mom stopped me. Her plans for her new garden didn't include my tunnel. Besides, she said, it will collapse and crush me.

But I could dig a deep tunnel under our backyard, to my nest in the Presidio, safe from earthquakes, cave-ins, Soviet missiles and any dangers. I wouldn't need to dig to China; simply a few cozy rooms, my pad in the dark, damp earth. Me and the earthworms. Nothing too fancy. I was a kid, not Bilbo Baggins. I'd build it solid, though, for a safe, warm chamber of refuge. My tunnel would wind through the earth with the worms and bugs decomposing and multiplying, their buried eggs preparing to hatch. Camouflage the entry with shrubs, and dirt, and pebbles.

They might uncover the entrance, the fake entrance that is, with the right maps and if they have stick-to-it-tiveness. Move the dirt concealed hatch and descend. I'd install hand and footholds for the climb, except mine made of wood, not a manhole's steel. But at the bottom, they'd run into dead ends, blocked passageways. Because I hid the actual doorway. And, if they discovered the hidden cat-door, they'd be too bulky to fit. If they squeezed through, my H.Q. hid deeper. Nobody checks for a secret door hidden in a wall of books, buried underground.

But, say they open the secret entrance. What lies in the centre, in the dark, hidden guts of the guts? Well, me, of course. Likely, I'd be making a Monte Cristo sandwich in the well-appointed underground kitchen, with stocked pantries. (Well, a little like Bilbo's.) A Monte Cristo with strawberry jam and sour cream on the side. Lots of cushions stack against the living room walls to get comfy. They'd hear the Contours singing "Do You Love Me" from the record player. Join me on the pillows digging the Supremes or Sam Cooke. And 33s: *The Freewheeling Bob Dylan*, Lightnin' Hopkins on Folkways, Paul Desmond. Sure, I'd fix a sandwich for guests.

And play a game of chess. I'd accommodate a chessboard in my subterranean sanctuary, with simple wooden pieces and a pressed cardboard board. Chess is hard. Still, it's fun, win or lose, when a visitor wants a game. What else? I mentioned books. Oh, and a toy train. In case I needed to chugga chugga choo choo out of town.

But anyways, nobody could unearth me in my secret brown sanctuary, warm and safe with the worms in the roots, and the deep insects. Me and dead leaves and live seeds shelter here and remain here for our moment to emerge from the earth.

Earthworms, if you think about it, are mostly guts. Guts with primitive light sensors. I mean, from an evolutionary standpoint, worms existed long before us. Earthworms dug their holes across and around backyard tunnels forever. Guts sense where light shines because mucus surrounds guts. Exposed to light, mucus dries up and the guts die.

So the gut-worms grew nerve receptors to distinguish light from dark, that became eyes and a brain to wonder and contemplate worms. But the guts are the real brains and pilots of the operation. The guts steer the ship. We started as guts who grew legs to vamoose or flippers to swim. And they grew spines, bones, and hair, hands to snag food, and teeth to munch things into the guts and hopes and dreams of little kids. Sorry to be a party pooper, but, too bad for me, my guts hurt.

## Why Mom moved so much, 1963

I appeared fine — chubby little Jewish boy. Your tummy making trouble? Well, look in the mirror. Mom and Dad's own problems, and dealing with Stephen's increasing troubles, absorbed their energy and focus. They didn't fret about big brother, Peter. They provided piano lessons while he continued to excel at sports and academics and began performing publicly.

When feeling well herself, Mom drove me to doctors, hunting for one who could heal me. There and back, in her 1958 Rambler Cross Country, she pointed out her childhood homes, schools attended, hideouts. We drove around San Francisco, side-by-side in her station wagon time machine seeking answers to the puzzles of my stomach and her past.

By then, in the early 1960s, we'd moved three times. I went to a lot of schools. Through the sixties and seventies, I attended five elementary schools, two junior highs, two high schools. Mom moved far more.

Every second block she'd share a memory of a place she lived or a school she attended. "We rented an apartment on this street awhile." "I attended that school for a few months." "Oh look, I hid out there in the winter of '38."

---

Coming back from a doctor's office on Nob Hill, we stopped at an intersection near Roosevelt Junior High. She stared out the window at every passer-by on Arguello Boulevard. No doctors in sight. She's somewhere else. Lost in her story or memory. Mom checked every face crossing her sight, searching for someone, not a doctor.

A honking and shout broke her memory. "C'mon lady, kick off time."

She started the Rambler, smiled, "'How poor are they that have not patience!' I should take you to see *Othello*."

"Ma, I saw *Othello*." Perched next to you. Like now.

"Down there, ol' Keith, Geary Boulevard, my grandmother's place. She'd serve Hungarian royal dinners or I stayed there when it became too rough at home."

"Too rough?"

"Oh, Joe charmed birds out of trees, dear, but he loved the bottle." Glancing at me while driving, "And your grandmother is such a delicate flower, requiring constant tending. Exhausting taking care of her, then fetching Joe from the alley behind the Little Shamrock. On school nights, I needed a quiet place to study."

Grandpa Joe, I never met, but the grandmother part rang true. When we visited her in Sacramento, she required constant tending. She called Dad, Robbie, demanding this or that. "Robbie, you and Big Peter move this over here; I'm much too weak." Lying on her old-country *dívány*, "adjust the light, would you? It's in my eyes." Then, "Robbie, mix me a cocktail." But the drink tastes too sour, or too thin, or too who knows. Delicate, blue-haired California flower. Sure, but c'mon, Mom, that's not the whole story. Nobody runs away from home to study.

## Swallow a wire, Hospital room, 1964

The fevers, diarrhea, and vomiting persisted, leading my parents and doctors to believe my illness existed, not all in my head. They hospitalized me for testing. Doctor after doctor came to my bed. They pressed on my stomach, listened with their stethoscope, or gently massaged under my chin with thoughtful expressions. One or two even looked compassionate, concentrating on my answers, shaking their heads. Others didn't examine me, instead scanned papers on a clipboard hanging by my bed and spoke in secret doctor-code. They poked and prodded — proctosigmoidoscopy, barium enema, Upper G.I. Series. To extract bone marrow, they drilled into my ribs.

To fetch a biopsy of my innards, they tried something new: I swallowed a wire with metal teeth at one end. A plunger stuck out the other end to activate the teeth. The teeth end would travel down to my gut and fetch a biopsy.

Here's the plan: I would swallow this chewing gum size ball with teeth, attached to a wire. The ball will somehow travel past the epiglottis barrier over the windpipe and into my esophagus. Down the esophagus and through the lower esophageal sphincter into the stomach. With no way to direct it, the ball is supposed to pass through the stomach, travel across the pyloric sphincter and into my small intestine. All the while it pulled a wire coming out my throat, with a plunger at the other end. Once it arrives at a promising location, the doctors plunge the plunger, the teeth chomp off a piece of tissue. They'd pull it out and examine what they found. Meanwhile, the wire at the top scraped back and forth across my throat.

Every hour, they scanned to follow its descent. They pressed a rubber disc into my abdomen at painful angles, probing for the ball's location. At the same time, I gagged and choked and tried to swallow the wire. After forty-eight hours of this futile torment, I pulled it out in tears. It barely travelled a few inches into my throat.

The doctor stared blankly at papers on a clipboard. "Just as well. Unlikely to descend deep enough."

The tests came back inconclusive. They'd run out of tests. After a week, they sent me home without a diagnosis. They didn't say the symptoms were imaginary.

Not crazy, but not normal. More than sleepy, I often couldn't keep my eyes open. My stomach felt tender and hot most of the time. Cramps often woke me. I suffered from both constipation and diarrhea — that's crazy.

But nothing appeared wrong — a normal chubby kid with fervent blue eyes. To the outside, I looked fine. So, fatigue wasn't my problem, laziness was. My problem, it seemed obvious, lay not in disease, pain, or my stomach. My problem remained me — careless, unfocused, lazy, irresponsible, unrealistic, unimportant, unwanted, unwantable.

# Not a New Disease

## A barber and a midwife

MEDICAL HISTORIANS CALL THE German doctor Wilhelm Fabry (1560–1634) the father of modern surgery. At age ten, Fabry's father died, so the family sent him to train as a barber's assistant. In those days, barbers performed medical procedures, including blood-lettings and surgeries. They treated burns, fractures, even tumours and ulcers. Apothecaries supplied potions and elixirs, but were not entitled to prescribe. Above the barber-surgeons and apothecaries loomed the physicians, who "having university degrees saw themselves as the top of the pyramid, walking about in cap and gown and spouting wisdom in Latin."[8]

In his twenties, Fabry served as a medical apprentice to the Duke of Cleves. Unlike other barber-surgeons, he voraciously studied anatomy, medicine, and dissections. Fabry promoted the novel idea that surgeons should and could understand human anatomy. He performed roughly six-hundred autopsies to apply anatomy and science to healing.

Fabry and his wife, Marie Colinet, invented surgical tools and methods for amputations and treating cancers. He'd successfully saved a six-month-old infant dying from a bowel blockage (pyloric stenosis). The medical establishment considered any obstruction below the stomach to be incurable. The baby survived to lead a full life. Many modern surgical techniques are based on their methods.

Originally a mid-wife, Colinet came up with new ways to do eye surgery, treat burns, and widen the cervix during difficult births. She performed the first recorded cesarean section where mother and baby both survived. She also bore eight children of her own through two outbreaks of the plague. With all her innovations, you might expect Colinet would be considered the mother of modern surgery. Nope.

## Morgue, Lausanne Hospital, 1612

Dr. Wilhelm Fabry roamed amongst three tables, adjusting feeble oil lamps. Morning light came in through a tall window on the east wall. A teenage boy's body lay prone on the largest table. The boy passed away the previous day, after complaints of stomach pain and diarrhea, two floors above where Fabry and a nun prepared to autopsy.

"The child's belly burned to my touch," said the nun who'd cared for the boy. "The Devil's bloody flux." A lifetime changing bedpans and bandages of the sick, the wounded, and dying showed on her lined face.

For weeks, she'd kept notes of his fevers emanating from his stomach, not his head. Now the Lord took the boy, she'd assist Fabry as she could. In truth though, she remained suspicious of his strange tools, his drawings, and his books.

Fabry needed her aid to determine the cause of the boy's death. This sister attended the doomed boy in life. Despite her superstition and ignorance, she provided the boy comfort and would now inform their examination.

The two positioned in front of the body. Fabry questioned her about the boy's bloody stools, urine, pulse, fevers. He recorded her responses in a notebook on the second table, glancing from his notebooks to the body.

The nun answered, "The Lord brought the child home for the Lord's own purpose."

Fabry paused, stifling his impatience, lips parted. He turned his attention from the body to the living woman. She had the spare look of one who'd spent a lifetime tending to the worst of human misery, while subservient to arrogant doctors and the prioress.

Fabry nodded slowly. "Sister, we can not fathom the Lord's purpose. Today, we behold and record His work."

The nun scrutinized his tools arranged on the third table, disapproval showing in her narrowed eyes and upturned nose. The church no longer banned dissections and autopsies. Still, she believed the boy's slight chance of entrance to heaven would not improve by showing up carved in pieces. She whispered to Fabry: opening the child would reveal demons inside stoking hell's furnaces.

She stepped back from the knives, saws, chisel, retractor, dilator. Fabry and Colinet designed most of the implements themselves.

On the second table, he'd placed a worn woodblock print of Andreas Vesalius's meticulous internal organ drawings. Next to the print he arranged his and Colinet's own notes and drawings from previous cases. The nun's case notes and hospital records also lay open on the table.

"Come, Sister. Let's admit God's light." The two adjusted the table with the body to maximize the light from the window. He noted the time and began his examination of the boy's limbs, head, skin, every inch of the outsides. Rigor mortis had passed. With the nun's aid, he flipped the body face up. He opened the mouth, examined gums, the tongue, under the tongue, the teeth. On the mouth's roof he found tiny abscesses.

The examination continued on each finger and toe. Several finger joints showed damage, but he detected no indication of injury. A mystery. As far as Fabry knew, children did not contract rheumatism.

The time came to examine inside.

An unmistakable stink met Fabry's incision of the belly. The nun covered her eyes, not her nose. Afraid of seeing the tiny demons and their tiny furnaces? Fabry knew nothing of germs, but he recognized the foul sepsis aroma. He again noted the time. They'd been at it for over an hour. The stench did not emanate from decay. Death occurred too recently. The internal organs had rotted, not decomposed. By their appearance, he guessed for several weeks.

He found more wrong. The anatomy baffled Fabry. He found intestinal structures missing or out of place, the bowel fibrous and riddled with holes. He searched vainly for the boy's cecum, a pouch-like structure at the colon's end. The ileum, a much narrower, longer tube, should extend out from the pouch.

Fabry halted the autopsy, swallowing, rubbing his hands. He examined the drawings, both Vesalius's pioneering masterworks and those he and his wife prepared. He examined their copious notes from other autopsies. The drawings and the boy's viscera differed. Where hid the cecum, normally at the end of the large bowel? The appendix also remained concealed.

The day prior, a complicated labour called his wife away. Once delivered, she'd need at least five hours by fast carriage along Lake Geneva to return to Lausanne and their children. Fabry's face lightened. Marie will save the mother's life and attend a new life. Meanwhile, here is this boy's mystery and death. A colon has a cecum. But where?

"Sister, adjust that lamp. We need more light here." Slowly, Fabry resumed, making detailed notations of everything he touched or observed. He recorded everything, so that later, once his wife returned, she'd help understand what killed the boy. Using the retractor, he eased organs aside, opening the view. Still, no cecum. He needed to incise the organs.

He selected a pair of dissecting scissors with angled blades his wife designed for her eye surgeries. Using the small, round tipped scissors he carefully dissected the distended, inflamed, bloody ileum. Instead of smooth and elastic, the ileum felt fibrous, rough and pocked. There. Finally, he found the missing organ in the wrong place, an impossible place. Holes perforated the bloody, inflamed cecum, nearly beyond recognition.

The gut had twisted into itself. The cecum lay contorted inside the boy's ileum, making movement of food or waste impossible. The boy's intestines inverted themselves, turned inside out; his guts revolted against themselves. They were not pink, soft, or hale. No demons. The boy's own body attacked itself. Confusion became horror. Fabry shook his head, left and right. What caused this monstrous self-violence?

Nothing made sense, not the premature rheumatism, the swollen, pus filled abscesses in the boy's mouth, the scrambled innards. The mystery deepened. How did he die? With rotting organs and bowels twisted inside out, how in God's name had the child lived; what inner force kept him alive?

Over the following centuries, other autopsies found similar horrors.

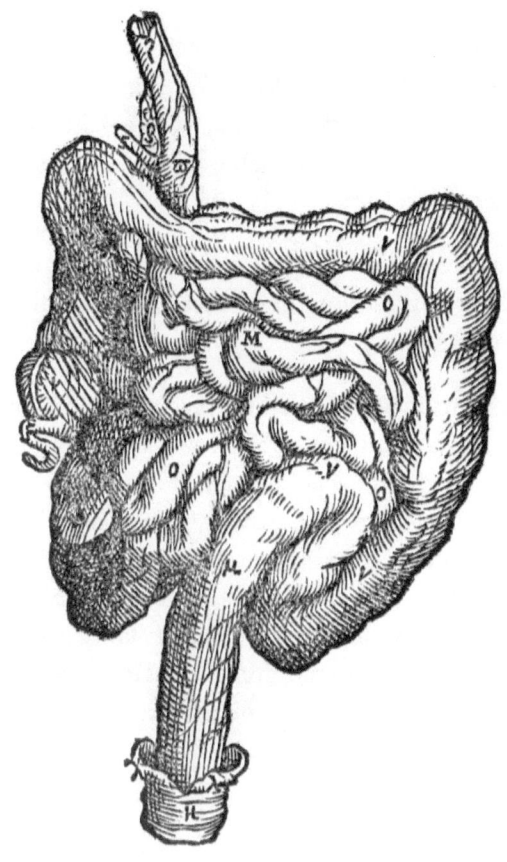

*(Wikimedia Commons Image licensed under the Creative Commons Attribution 4.0 International license at https://creativecommons.org/licenses/by/4.0/legalcode.)*

Dr. Fabry may have used a woodblock print of this 1543 drawing by Andreas Vesalius. Normally, the large bowel, 'V' on the drawing, terminates with the pouch on the left, the cecum. The worm-like structure just below is the appendix. Vesalius did not draw precisely the terminal ileum, the end of the small intestine, 'O', where it meets the cecum. The shady area between the cecum and small intestine approximates its location. A smooth sphincter muscle separates the 3-4 cm long, 1.25–1.5 inches terminal ileum and the cecum. In the boy's autopsy, Fabry found the cecum inside the terminal ileum.

## The death of a bigamous lady of charm and wealth

In 1859, the London police charged and convicted Dr. Thomas Smethurst of poisoning his second wife, Isabella Bankes. Bankes, "a bigamous lady of charm and some means,"[9] suffered in life "with persistent sickness and diarrhoea."[10] Smethurst was headed for the gallows. Fortunately the medical profession rallied behind him.

The authorities ordered a second autopsy. One doctor administered arsenic, the suspected poison, to dogs, then compared the effect on the animals to Bankes' autopsy.

Another doctor testified: "The intestines presented appearance of excessive inflammation, and the lining membrane was almost certainly destroyed. There was likewise blood in the stomach."[11] Thirty eminent physicians examined Bankes' body and the evidence. They agreed Bankes did not die from poison but disagreed on the actual cause of death, other than inflamed, bloody bowels. Bankes had been pregnant and one doctor said she died as a result. Other doctors said dysentery killed her; another, starvation. They wrote a petition to the Home Secretary.[12] Smethurst received a pardon. Forensic doctors and the sleuths who cherish history and mysteries argue the case to this day. Most conclude Bankes died from Crohn's.

## Freud, CD, and lobotomies

In the early twentieth century, more suffering, more baffling cases, and more hideous deaths. Autopsies found bowels hard as rock and packed with blood. Sigmund Freud declared the cause to be "psychic colitis." Rage without normal avenues for expression, Freud surmised, would channel inward and scorch the bowel.[13] The medical establishment authorized prefrontal lobotomies as treatment.

In 1932 Dr. Burrill Crohn and two other doctors at New York's Mt Sinai Hospital identified regional ileitis as a distinct disorder.[14] Throughout his long life and career, Crohn resisted the later renaming of the ailment to Crohn's disease. Dr. Crohn was the only person at a conference in Prague who objected to using the name "Crohn's disease." The officials ruled him to be out of order and now the disorder carries his name.[15]

Four centuries ago, Dr. Fabry searched in vain for the cause of another boy's self-destruction. The twentieth-century medical profession assigned a name to the affliction, Crohn's disease (CD), but its cause remains a mystery to this day.

---

When my suffering started in the 1960s, the medical profession still thought emotions or personality caused CD. Pioneer gastroenterologist Dr. Joseph B. Kirsner fought compassionately for seventy-five years to relieve the misery of CD. Dr. Kirsner wrote: "Psychiatric precepts during the 1930s, 1940s, and 1950s emphasized an 'ulcerative colitis personality', described as 'immaturity of the patient, indecisiveness, over-dependence, and inhibited interpersonal relationships,' together with critical emotional events including the loss of a loved one, feelings of social rejection, and 'maternal dominance'."[16]

In Freud's footsteps, research up to the sixties focussed on finding a psychogenic cause for ulcerative colitis. Dr. Crohn's research in the 1930s established CD as a separate disease from ulcerative colitis. Still, most research lumped them together. Research claimed patients "couldn't cope, giving up"; "diarrhea is substituted for real accomplishment."[17] In the nineties, an associate of my family doctor, who'd never examined me, said, in passing, "Your personality type tends to Crohn's." It's all in your head, kid.

## Who we are

About 270 thousand Canadians (2018)[18] and 3 million US adults (2015)[19] are diagnosed with CD or ulcerative colitis. The sheer suffering is staggering. People's mouths surgically removed. People crippled by Crohn's Related Arthritis (CRA). Young people wear ostomy bags to collect their waste. A seventy-year-old man lost his arm to Crohn's related gangrene. Prior to the gangrene, he'd been twenty-six years symptom free.

Amputations are rare. Gangrene from Crohn's, pyoderma gangrenosum, is less rare and, if identified early, treatable. I've had gangrene from Crohn's twice.

We seem fine. If you meet someone with Crohn's who is thin, do not assume they have found a successful diet. More likely, they are starving to death.

In "What It's Like Living with Crohn's," Katherine Chang wrote, "Although someone with Crohn's may not look sick, trust me when I say it very likely took every bit of strength and will for that person to get out the door."[20]

A child's experience from the Boston Children's Hospital Experience Journal: "I lost a lot of weight, I wasn't growing, I had constant diarrhea, and anything I ate went directly through my system. And I was tired; I slept the majority of the day away. I remember thinking that the most mundane tasks were virtually impossible for me. Like how I was going to get to school, which was a couple of blocks away. How was I going to muster up the energy to walk there?"[21]

And, something else, impossible for me to talk about: an underlying sense that my identity didn't belong to me. The other kids in school were the "real" students. Each time we moved, I arrived at my new class in a new school late. The students sat in their seats. They knew which seats were theirs, how to sit, how to play and study and be kids. They were the actual students. On a good day, I donned my kid mask and faked it, performing an act.

This sense of being unreal couldn't come from my illness. This performance thing must have been in my head, even if the pain in my stomach proved real.

Turns out, a connection exists between developing identity and being ill. Children living with chronic disease often suffer stilted development, physically, socially, *and* developmentally. Children and adults with diseases of the immune system experience a kind of self-identity loss. All people put on masks and personas, appropriate for different circumstances. Research is showing that many with autoimmune disease are impersonating *themselves*. We are pretending, not just at being an employee, a lover, a citizen, we are pretending at being people.

# The Festival

**Siddhartha's story, Kingdom of Koshala, 451 BCE**

WHEN SIDDHARTHA BECAME NINE, his father and step-mother took him to their clan's annual plowing festival. His father decided the time had arrived to train the boy for his future responsibilities leading the Shakya clan. To teach Siddhartha to stay close to the earth, the source of the clan's fortunes.

After planning and labour for weeks, the day arrived for the festival celebrating the commencing of the annual growing cycle. Plowing also culminated the toil of manuring, tilling, crop husbandry and rotation, and irrigation. The nobles, members of the warrior class, dressed in their finest. Flags waved. *Mahouts* paraded a massive war elephant festooned with banners and topped with a riding carriage. The court musicians tuned their harps and veenas. Tables creaked under mountains of delicacies and drink. Siddhartha's father, the clan's head, arranged for soldiers to keep beggars and thieves well away.

Before the festivities, Brahmin priests recited passages from the Vedas. They said prayers for fine weather and a bountiful harvest. Then, they preached about the benefits of animal sacrifice, and how to behave properly according to the caste system. This was nature's order. A priest pronounced: "As a man has a head to reason, so society has Brahmins to instruct. As a man has hands to toil and craft, society has warriors, the Kshatriyas to rule."

But listening to the preaching bored the children. The royal children liked entertainment and treats, not sermons. The court ladies and their servants led the restless children away, to not disturb the rituals. Away from the sermons, jugglers, snake charmers, and a puppet show entertained them.

Except Siddhartha. Alone, he meandered around the festival grounds, fascinated by the behaviour of the priests and the revellers. The air filled with the smells of incense, perfume, and pigs roasting on bonfires. Stilt walkers paraded between stalls, their bodies painted in white and red. Some were dressed as women, others as animals and heavenly birds, *kimnaras*. They were accompanied by third gender *kinnar* drummers and flutists playing music of the Koshalan kingdom. Festival labourers rushed in last-minute preparations, barking orders to cooks and entertainers. The birds overhead flew in graceful, enchanting patterns. Bullocks strained, chained to plows. Insects crawled at his feet and buzzed in his face. A marvellous day.

The event fascinated yet perplexed him. Those three men: the Brahmin preaches; the nobleman heeds; behind the nobleman stands his retainer, poised to serve. The three came here to this festival, the Brahmin to preach, the noble to hear, the servant to serve. Why? Why must each man act according to these exact roles? What if the servant was heard, the Brahmin was humble, and the nobleman helped others?

Siddhartha knew the answers people told. His tutors told stories of endless lifetimes of karma. Others said a wise and powerful god decided. Siddhartha loved stories, hearing them and telling them and making them. Why did one story carry more truth than others?

A child's questions. Questions that would trouble Siddhartha for decades to come. Questions about roles, purpose, and misery bothered Siddhartha like a nagging toothache.

His father expected him to learn lessons that day. He agreed. He learned much more here at the festival than repeating dogma, seated for hours across from tutors.

## The worms scream

Finally finishing, the priests told the attendants where to find temporary altars and donation collection tables. The plowing ceremony began.

Siddhartha's father wore a ceremonial cotton robe, dyed with madder herb and an upper garment from the hide of a spotted deer. A sacred thread hung over his shoulder. He passed his banyan wood staff to a servant, who handed him a whip in return. He took the handles of a decorated six bullock plow. He cracked the whip, and the animals pulled. Father furrowed one row to applause and music and general gaiety. The bulls looked tortured. They endured the whip for the ceremony's sake and for the sake of growing food for humans. In young Siddhartha's eyes, one living being suffered for another's pleasure.

After father's first ceremonial turn, the real plowmen set to labour. Their half-naked, sun-baked bodies glistened with sweat. The royals ate and danced and enjoyed the festivities.

Siddhartha wandered the field. The plows turned up the earth, and everything in the earth, including insects and earthworms. The worms wriggled in the sun, desperate to crawl back underground before their mucus coating dried and they died. Many didn't return home under the dirt, their lifeless bodies strewn across the ridges and furrows. The plows cutting through the earth sliced through other worms and bugs. Small birds flocked near the rows to feast on the insects. Hawks circled overhead, then dove to capture and feast on the small birds.

Siddhartha considered what he'd observed. To survive, another died. Every life ends in death, both eaters and eaten. And every being's life depends on another's dying. Siddhartha imagined the worms' screams, the captured birds' cries, the whips' burns, cracking on the oxen's backs.

Whether a creature lived in misery or fear or pleasure was not random. Their destiny of suffering or joy did not depend on virtue, or wisdom, or righteousness. Every creature's station determined their fate, not behaviour or choices or divine intervention. Worms or oxen, or servants or nobles or peasants; each lived a very different life. The cycle of life, yes. But he also observed a cycle of life and death and privilege and disadvantage.

## What puppets imagine

He joined the other children in games, shooting clay marbles and spinning tops. His younger cousin, Devadatta, won most of the games, but that's fine. Win or lose, Siddhartha enjoyed playing.

To Siddhartha's joy, the *mahouts* offered him the first ride on the elephant.

The chance to mount the grand animal excited him. His father's position granted him the first ride. To his disappointment, his playmates could not join him in the spacious howdah.

The magnificent creature kneeled, and he climbed up the right foreleg. He felt like he was in the forest, climbing an enormous tree trunk. The skin was rough and wrinkly, and felt like bark to his touch. One *mahout* lifted him into the howdah carriage and secured him with a golden rope around his waist.

Siddhartha wore a green and yellow knee-length tunic over strong canvas pantaloons. His step-mother had tied his topknot with a bright royal blue ribbon. The *mahouts* had washed the splendid animal for the festival. It smelled of must and musk and the forest, covered by soap nuts and acacia.

Thrilled, the boy looked out from the howdah for his friends. Adults and children cheered, "Siddhartha, Lord Siddhartha, as noble as a prince!"

From the elephant's back, he took in the festive scene. Nobles feasted, the plowmen strained at their labours, the musicians and entertainers performed. He watched the puppeteers from above and behind, pulling the puppets' strings. The angle blocked his view of the puppets themselves. He imagined the puppets as living beings imagining themselves. The puppet people imagined they lived real lives and made actual choices, unaware of the strings and their hidden masters.

Further out, the soldiers marched in the sun at the fields' edges and, beyond the soldiers, lingered the poor. Each person behaved differently and others treated them differently because of their station. And somehow, in some way, he struggled to grasp, they were all one.

## Prayers did not help

His father and step-mother gathered him at the end of the festival so the family could pray at the altars and make offerings. "Father, Mommy Mausi, the priests' prayers did not aid the worms."

His step-mother leaned towards the boy. "What do you mean, young Lord?"

"The worms hurt and died." That got his father's attention. He feared his son might quit home to seek a spiritual life and forsake his duties as the heir to the Shakyas. Times grew difficult. The clan required leadership, foresight, and strength to avoid being swept away by history.

He adopted a wise, kindly tone. "Son, I brought you to the festival for the sake of our clan's future, not for daydreams. The worms suffer because of evil acts they committed in past lives, their karma. Your tutors will instruct you in detail."

"No, Father, not karma. The worms suffer because the plow broke their home or chopped them. I saw their deaths."

His step-mother knelt to his level, eye to eye. She'd loved him, raised him as her own child since infancy. Her adoring gaze met Siddhartha's. Then she rose and regarded his father. He cherished his son, truly and terribly. "The dear boy's imagination, Lord. In the future, his creativity will serve you and the clan well."

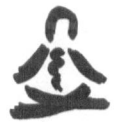

# "No team wants you."

## Sick, isolated, angry, Los Angeles, 1966

WE'D MOVED AGAIN, THIS time from San Francisco to Los Angeles. The further south Dad's career took us, the more miserable the family became; the sicker and angrier I became.

Teachers had no reason to be sympathetic. They didn't understand. I couldn't go to a new teacher at a new school and proclaim, "Hi, I will need to use the bathroom a lot because of my stomach. But I can't bring a note from a doctor. Doctors don't understand what I have or if anything is really wrong." I missed school from fatigue, pain, and hospital stays. When uncertain about controlling my body, I skipped school, becoming more cut off from others.

## Elysian Fields Baseball Park

I got on a Little League team. Too short and slow, but my arm threw like a rifle. Coach said the team needed a back-up catcher or third base. With my arm, I'd throw out runners. I mostly rode the bench. Rode the bench and heckled the opposing team.

On the bench, my mouth roared. Badgered the opposition pitchers, hitters, their coaches, mothers. My way to be part of the team, contribute. I got the other side's attention and pissed them off. My teammates finally told me to shut up. The unwritten rule: if they attack our player, everyone on our team defends him. They didn't want to protect the obnoxious, back-up bench warmer if a brawl started.

I never missed a game, but missed a couple of practices and left one game early because of cramps. That day, the pain doubled me over, like baseballs popping against my belly while my insides were being squeezed and twisted. The team jersey brushing against my burning stomach chafed. The pain continued, familiar but unbearable. I couldn't even sit the bench.

---

Before the 1967 season began, coach sat me down. "We are going to cut you. Your arm is strong. You play ball smart, to make up for your lack of size and speed and skill. Regardless, no team wants you. The other boys are growing stronger, taller, faster. No time-outs for the toilet."

I stood no chance to be normal, try normal stuff. I didn't belong to any team. Kids my age grew. I got weaker and softer. No school group activities for me. Lying in bed, I played baseball on the ceiling, the walls' corners forming the diamond, moving imaginary teammates in and out.

## Three Strangers, 1967

One evening, Pete came home with three new friends around his age — late teens, early twenties. They dressed conventionally, unlike his fellow musicians or Steve and my hippie friends. I shuffled to the living room to meet them. They politely introduced themselves and the three spoke, smiling and animated. The drummer and bass player who came for rehearsal did neither.

The young woman's eyes twinkled as she gazed directly at me, then Stephen. She smiled easily. "I'm Nancy. You're Pete's brothers? I'm delighted to meet you." As if, in an impossible universe, Pete told her marvellous tales of his little brothers. She wore a knee-length orange skirt and a plain white top with her bright, generous expression.

They said they were members of a Buddhist group, and that they recited the title of the Lotus Sutra, Nam-myoho-renge-kyo. One man, wearing wire-rimmed glasses and a corduroy jacket, turned to me. "You know, the law of cause and effect." I didn't know. I'd never heard of any of this.

Pete took them into his room. From our bedroom, Stephen and I overheard their chanting. What a sound, over and over, Nam-myoho-renge-kyo. Incense aroma floated from his room. Incense. Groovy.

They came out. Mom stopped them from leaving, arranging the three at the dining room table. Mom didn't smile, but inquired if they needed anything. Nancy asked for a glass of water. I fetched it, then stationed myself next to Stephen. Would they conduct a debate or an interrogation? Hopefully, Pete was in trouble. Nancy emptied the entire glass in one enthusiastic gulp. I leapt to refill her glass, and she responded with a bubbly smile.

"Tell us about yourselves," Mom directed.

Stephen gave me the slightest nod of approval as I plunked back next to him. Behind the three, lights of the LA basin glimmered through the picture window and brown-grey smog. They explained what they called the basics of Buddhism. The guy in the corduroy jacket spoke earnestly, leaning forward from his seat and smiling. "Life and environment are one, a system. If life changes, its environment adjusts. By chanting Nam-myoho-renge-kyo, we tap that potential from within. We enlarge our lives on a fundamental level. It's a human revolution. This individual revolution will contribute to world peace."

Pete said he joined their group after attending their meetings. News to me, but it sounded as though he'd already spoken with Mom and Dad.

Dad tapped his pipe, quizzed them, sceptical. "I've done research into Soka Gakkai. Isn't your group controversial in Japan? I read Soka Gakkai gained popularity among people of questionable backgrounds, Tokyo bar maids. And what about the involvement in politics I read about?"

Nancy turned squarely towards Dad as he spoke. He fussed with his pipe. Her eyes moved with his to the pipe, tracking his gaze. I glanced at Stephen, check it out. She's encouraging him.

Pete: "Father, they're improving their lives."

Nancy: "Dr. Robinson, our organization will always be on the side of regular people. Our founder, a teacher, died in prison, opposing the Japanese military during World War II. Our goal is lasting world peace." Her words came evenly with strength: "I have asthma, getting worse and worse with the smog. I thought I would have to drop out of school, Cal State Northridge. Then I started practising. The attacks are under control. I breathe much better now, I'm determined to make the Dean's list. I'm studying hard and my breathing is clearer."

Bob jumped in, speaking quicker than Nancy: "I'm a musician, rhythm guitar. Rock, don't understand Pete's jazz. My best friend died last year in Vietnam. It hurt so much."

Bob slowed. "Damn, it tormented me. I was lost. Couldn't play. Couldn't eat. Would I starve or go nuts? So messed up, angry and confused, I started doing drugs. Then more drugs. When I set the alarm for the middle of the night to wake up and get high, I figured out drugs weren't helping me, or my friend, or the war. A girl told me about chanting."

Bob's gaze landed on Mom. "No offense, Mrs. Robinson, but she interested me more than Buddhism." Mom appeared caring, not offended. She shrugged, then gave herself a slight hug, her eyelids drooped. Bob kept going: "A girlfriend might make me feel better. I started chanting. Turned out she didn't want to be my girlfriend. She wanted me to be happy. Gradually I began coming back. Playing again. Forming a band."

Bob's voice lowered, slowed. Focused and determined. "Now I know how I'm going to spend my life. Create music for peace, for all those who die in the insanity of war." This guy leaned forward, his eyes shone. His sincerity and passion surprised me; he spoke without any cool, jive musician-speak.

Not a debate. Although I didn't get them, these people spoke from their hearts, genuine. Dad seemed more satisfied. To Dad, Pete joined a movement, not converted to a religion. That's Dad.

Mom, although fascinated by Asian culture, remained doubtful. But Peter didn't take drugs, didn't drink, and the top music schools chased him to apply. He wasn't their problem. Other problems occupied Mom and Dad.

Mom addressed Bob. "I'm very sorry for your friend. What a waste, a horrible, horrible waste. We are fighting to end this war of aggression." She then switched to Pete: "It's your choice," she said, "as long as you keep your grades up."

None of the talk meant much to me. Didn't do drugs, other than marijuana, and that didn't count. School was okay; no intention of dropping out. Music will not end war. The Buddhism talk, the chanting — made no sense. These people are crazy if they believe chanting will end a war. At the same time, I desired their optimism and strength. I distrusted the peace talk; still it got my attention. I yearned for peace, inside and out. Anyway, religion was stupid and what Pete did, who cares? Nothing to do with me. Stephen split before they finished. I stayed and listened.

# The Swan

A FEW YEARS AFTER the plowing ceremony, Siddhartha and other royal children romped in the forest outside of Kapilavastu. Siddhartha's younger cousin, a handsome lad named Devadatta, carried a bow and quiver full of arrows. The broadleaf forest was a swell place to practice archery, show off his skills, and, with luck, impress the girls. A fine archer, Devadatta delighted in demonstrating his talents.

The children had reached that in-between age. They still played children's games, tag and hiding games (*chhupan chhupai*), but started becoming curious about each other.

Most of the girls ignored Siddhartha. Too broody. He held odd ideas and spent hours observing ant colonies or talking to servants and goatherds. Most of the girls enjoyed parcheesi (*pachisi*) and hopscotch or dress-up with their aunties' clothes and baubles.

## Forest, Upper Gangetic Plain, 447 BCE

Siddhartha delighted in the forest, becoming absorbed in its green and brown energy. He rolled over rotting leaves blanketing the forest floor. He climbed fresh growth erupting out of the decaying stumps of collapsed branches. The rich smell of fungi floated in the thick wind. Here, living beings battled to survive and all in continuous fading away.

Visiting the forest from season to season through his childhood, he noticed how it evolved. He found a naked rock in one season covered in moss the next. A pile of leaves grew into a bush the following year. Whatever entered the forest dissolved, absorbed by the forest, as if a giant mouth ingested all flora and fauna.

His childhood musings about life and death, futility and meaning, sharpened in the forest. The air carried the sounds of monkeys, wind, birds, the busyness of the place. The forest clamoured with activity, yet serene, so . . . itself. Behold, everything in the forest, from insects to animals to trees, is busy being born, growing, struggling to survive, and dying. All things in harmony and fierce competition.

If he explored deep enough into the forest, he might discover an ancient path to the ruins of a city that once held wisdom. But the forests of northern India held danger with bears, tigers, pythons, and bandits to kidnap a child of a noble family. So he and the others stayed close to well-travelled paths.

## Possession and belonging

The rustle of wings caught Siddhartha's attention. He glanced up past a clump of bushes to see a wedge of black and white swans take to the air. With grace and collective beauty, the wedge soared as one. Then he heard a horrible screech. One swan plunged out of the sky. The children scrambled in the direction it fell. Siddhartha found the fallen bird in a clearing. It lay unmoving, blood on its side. Nearby lay an arrow.

Siddhartha knelt by the bird's side, examining it. It seemed dead. He positioned himself cross-legged on the ground and lifted the bird onto his lap. Its broad chest barely moved.

A voice: "Hey drop that. It's mine." But Siddhartha's eyes and fingers stayed on the swan.

The other children arrived. Siddhartha continued examining the bird. The arrow scraped its side, tearing feathers. No bones seemed broken. The bird lay still under his fingers; without resistance, frozen, as if lifeless.

Devadatta, bow in hand, towered above Siddhartha on the ground. Devadatta said the bird belonged to him; he shot it. Others agreed with him, "Siddhartha, surrender the swan to Devadatta."

One, who considered himself learned, stroked his non-existent beard and deepened his voice. "Since days of yore, it has been thus: the reward of the hunt goes to the hunter."

One girl, Yasodhara, stepped out from the gathered children towards the two boys. "No, the bird belongs to the one who saved it." Some children agreed with Yasodhara, most with Devadatta.

Siddhartha stayed out of the debate. His fingers delicately moved over the animal's inert body, under the wing, along the breastbone. Dimly, the bird's heart beat, faint and slow. The bird remained completely immobile, but not dead. The injury seemed minor.

Devadatta grew frustrated. His voice held menace. "Give it to me. The trophy is mine. I mastered it." Siddhartha continued examining the swan, not glancing up at his cousin. Gently, he rotated the wing on the injured side, its motion unimpeded. Yet the bird remained motionless; its eyes blank, unblinking. The other children continued their debate, taking sides, as if in a contest. Yasodhara's sensitive gaze swept from Siddhartha's delicate fingers to the bird. She'd never noticed his unwavering eyes before, hazel under aristocratic brows.

He hadn't saved the animal; he knew that much. He tried to consider its perspective, uncover what happened. It flew free with its wedge. Then, without warning, the arrow struck, knocking it from flight and to the ground. Now, it lay injured in the arms of a creature five times its size. A giant. Of course it froze. He hadn't saved the bird; it became his captive.

"No," said Siddhartha, "Here is a free being, belonging only to itself. It is I who caused it to seem dead." He released his grip, opened his hands, and gave a gentle toss. The wings flapped, the swan alighted away.

In that moment, as the bird flew free, Yasodhara's heart was captured. She fell utterly in love with Siddhartha; how could she not? Greater than a wizard who resurrects the dead, he freed the bird to be itself. Not a magician, a liberator.

## Yasodhara chooses, Koliya clan home

That evening, Yasodhara spoke with her mother and father. She told them about Devadatta shooting the swan. She described how the children debated who possessed the swan, and how Siddhartha ignored the debate and concentrated on caring for the bird.

Her father said: "An interesting question of title. I wonder how a magistrate would rule in such a case. These are the kinds of questions Siddhartha will deal with when he leads his people. He should have paid more attention to the discussion. As a leader, he will need to consider the different points of view."

"Father, Siddhartha showed compassion and concentration. He examined the bird minutely. He considered the point of view of the injured animal. These are qualities I seek in a husband."

Husband? Wedding? Being doting parents of a thirteen-year-old, they expressed concerns. You are of the age to consider your future, dear, but we've heard troubling stories about this young man. He doesn't follow the traditional ways. They whisper he argues with his tutors and the priests. Young passion is one thing. Its fire burns bright, but will fade. Still, we must consider the future of two clans, the well-being of hundreds of families. The Shakyas may be in decline. Is he the leader to ensure their future prosperity or will he abandon you and us Koliyas, and the Shakyas on some spiritual folly?

Her mother probed, "What about the young Lord, darling? What holds his heart?"

Yasodhara replied, "My heart is set. I made my decision. I choose Siddhartha of the Shakyas."

Her father shook his head, defeated. "We will need to consult our family priest, the astrologers and diviners. Even with you choosing, we require a broker. I know his father well. The arrangements and negotiations will be arduous."

# This Is Real

At thirteen, physically sick and emotionally in rage, life hurt. My family tore itself apart. The world teetered on the brink of destructive revolutions. Inside and out, conflict and turmoil simmered or exploded.

The National Liberation Front and North Vietnamese armies launched their Tet offensive. The campaign made the final expulsion of the Americans inevitable. Czech citizens fought Soviet tanks sent to crush the Prague Spring. Ten days before the summer Olympics, troops and tanks in Mexico City attacked unarmed students, killing hundreds. At the Democratic National Convention in Chicago, police rioted. Every day fresh fires ignited. *Newsweek* magazine proclaimed 1968, "The Year That Changed Everything." Times changed. The world evolved, as the world does.

At school, I under-achieved, bored and often in trouble for causing disturbances or fighting. When not at school, I smoked dope with Stephen, attended anti-war demonstrations with Mom, and hung out at hippie love-ins.

On good days in LA, I explored Griffith Park and its observatory, hung out with artists at the Barnsdall Junior Arts Center. On sick days, bedridden and burning, I sang along to Bob Dylan. I studied large-scale maps of South Vietnam, charting battle and casualty reports, or I made elaborate tables of delegate counts for Chicago.

As I entered my teens, I transferred schools. Since I was the anonymous new kid, I could skip classes without repercussions. That idea didn't go as well as planned.

Could people be with each other to share laughter and pain? My family's nonconformity defined me — Mom and Dad's politics, their Beat

Generation rebelliousness, our secular Judaism. My early memories were of attending civil rights and anti-nuclear weapons protests. We marched and sang folk songs, became roused by speeches, met dedicated, fascinating people. Since our views differed from the norm, I related to the normal world by being against it. At one new school, a teacher requested I describe myself. My response, "different."

Wherever I was, home or school or with friends, I didn't belong. Nowhere felt safe, an intruder at home, a freak at school, barely tolerated by friends. I peered in windows, yearning to knock on their doors and shatter the doors, craving acceptance from those inside while wanting to destroy those inside.

No one explained why my stomach was on fire, why I wiped out exhausted so easily. No one and nothing to ask. One fear lay underneath, one question of questions with no-one to ask, not even myself: what if this never ends?

I took pride in my Jewish and Canadian roots. In fact, I knew little of either. A wistful longing pulled me towards my unexplored past. I craved a history simultaneously abandoned, magnetic, and an illusion.

## Not in my head, January 1968

My head felt hot and swimmy before I started towards home. Up the Loz Feliz hill, I hauled myself, my books, and my three-speed bike with high-rise handlebars and a banana seat. The rain didn't cool me. I paused a couple of times to steady myself. Got going again; now I needed to use the washroom. C'mon, fattie, a simple return home, you manage this every day. Sweat and steam rose, filling the hooded slicker and fogging my glasses. It took all my energy to stow my bike and struggle into the house for the toilet. Drained and dizzy, did I drop my textbooks? My head's still foggy. I clung to the door handle. Maybe I need a bowl of cereal. I slumped onto the toilet seat, head between my knees.

Stephen found me sometime later, on the floor. "Did you see in the toilet?"

"What? Yeah. No. I didn't see anything. Did I faint? Is that passing out? Where are my glasses?"

"It was full of blood. Pull up your pants. You're going to the hospital. A lot of blood, clumped and thick. What the fuck is wrong with you?"

They got me to the Kaiser Permanente Hospital, where I stayed three days. Not in my head. This isn't in my head. Not from eating too fast. This is serious. If it's not in my head and they don't figure out what's wrong, what's going to happen to me? I squeezed the bed railing until my knuckles went white and hand cramped. Actual blood. Am I going to shit blood until I die? Struggling for years to convince them this is real and, now, this is real. Nowhere to hide.

A pediatrician named Goldberg examined me. He must have my records, the doctors before him, the inconclusive tests. But he asked the same questions. Same answers, except one: My stomach is tender most of the time. The pain is real. I am tired all the time. I can't sleep. Cramps and going to the toilet wake me. I vomit, run fevers. But, passing blood, that's a first; what does that mean? What's wrong with me?

## Encephalitis or partying?

In her memoir, *Brain on Fire,* journalist Susannah Cahalan describes waking up to a hell on Earth: "At first there is just darkness and silence. 'Are my eyes open? Hello?' I can't tell if I am moving my mouth or if there is even anyone to ask." She could be describing a *lokāntarikā*, a lightless between-spaces hell. She is not in a mythological hell, but a human one, a New York mental hospital in 2009. Diagnosed with "partying too much" and a mood disorder, restrained with a straight jacket.

In fact, she had a rare form of encephalitis. "How many people throughout history suffered from my disease and others like it but went untreated?"[22]

An interviewer inquired, "What's it like to have a medical condition you can't explain?"

"It is utterly terrifying and lonely. I feel for people who don't have a proper diagnosis. It felt very claustrophobic. I was experiencing these emotions and feelings. I was hallucinating. You feel trapped inside your body."[23]

## Undiagnosed

"Undiagnosed diseases are common, affecting approximately 30 million Americans," reads a 2017 study of patients' narratives. One of the study's conclusions: "These narratives illustrate the chaos that coexists with being undiagnosed." Patient experiences include "searching for legitimacy of illness, uncertainty, fear, suffering, inability to consider a future or to make plans, and loss of control, self, or purpose."[24] Chaos coexists with being undiagnosed. Reading the study now, I realize how my family suffered the same chaos. Every time my parents considered me, they'd be reminded of their own uncertainties, fears, and loss of control. We tried desperately to strike our individual paths, yet remained bound in a knot without release. Today, too late, my heart goes out to them.

I lay in the bed at the Kaiser Permanente Hospital waiting for someone to announce what ailed me. Whatever my disorder, it didn't enjoy the benefit of a name. Real illness had names, horrible names, like muscular dystrophy, or polio, or epilepsy. I wasn't one of those handicapped kids. Having to go to the bathroom a lot couldn't really be considered a handicap. Well, not going out from fear I wouldn't find a bathroom became a sort of handicap. But not a real handicap like the kids who couldn't walk. Not going out because I might shit blood and pass out and maybe die, that's closer to a handicap.

Anyway, I look ok. I can still try what normal kids do. I don't wear a sign around my neck: "SICK, CONDITION UNKNOWN." None of their business. But something was wrong, not only my stomach. Something with me.

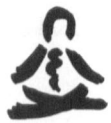

# Inflamed, Invisible

## Hidradenitis suppurativa

THE PEDIATRICIAN PUT ME on an iron supplement and released me from hospital, three days after I passed out. Day after day, my body tried to expel its intestines, attacking itself violently, destroying itself. No one saw; no one *could* see. And now this: passing out, passing blood.

Friends, teachers, doctors, Dad denied anything was wrong. I hated the pain, and since I wanted nothing to be wrong, nothing was wrong. With another sandwich and a nap, I'd be fine. Like the shadow people, in time, a light glowed from within me. Until then, I lived in between, in the dark.

Such were my innards in 1968. My outsides, no better. My family bickered and sulked. Once I asked a friend back over. "No, man, your place hurts."

---

Mom also suffered from a crappy auto-inflammatory disease. Hidradenitis suppurativa (HS) caused horrible, painful boils under her arms and breasts. The boils abscessed. They broke open, releasing a stinky pus, soiling her clothes. The boils reappeared in the same spots. As they healed over, inflamed tunnels formed beneath the surface. In the fifties, to relieve the endless boils, surgery removed her breast.

She often stayed in bed, weak, in pain, and resentful. I'd carry an Irish whiskey with soda and a lemon twist to her bed. No relief for her pains, but I'd receive a blessing, Irish or Hungarian. Lancing the abscesses required a doctor, often in hospital.

## The fight

The fight started at dinner. My parents fought a lot. They weren't shy. But this time, they didn't let up after dinner. They argued about Stephen, who'd left the house early. They argued about a bill becoming overdue when Mom didn't pay it because Dad misplaced it. Mom fancied a talk about a radio play she'd finished writing. Dad expected to talk about the smog, the heat, academic politics, LA traffic, no AC in the car. Issues vital at the time and meaningless now. Both dead now, beyond caring.

Dinner finished, a complicated vegetable casserole and lamb chops. Mom expressed her marvellous palate and innovation in every dish. She mastered all the skills expected of women in those days — gardening, of course; and cooking, and sewing Halloween costumes. As the years passed, her skills didn't diminish, but her resentments grew.

She resisted, in myriad ways, being identified, governed, and circumscribed by the roles for women of her time and culture. Dad's bottomless pit of wants sucked her limited energy and further limited her options. Two prisoners of lack of control, their unfulfilled needs plastered on the other and confused with love.

Of course, she resisted. After all, she'd parented Emma and Joe and still found her own way. You can expect me to both darn your socks and edit your papers, uncredited, but your expectations are not my identity. I will live my life.

I eavesdropped from across the room at the dining table, pretending to do homework. I'd cleared the dishes, the lamb fat on the plate congealed and Stephen's plate untouched. Now in the living room but visible from my seat in the dining room, they kept escalating. Shrunk behind the screen of my three-ring binder, I watched. With more bile, uglier, each wanting the other to hurt. Neither let go. Neither backed down. They couldn't quit.

The truth came out: Mom claimed the mastectomy proved unnecessary and blamed Dad. "You don't castrate a man for a boil, a skin disease."

"You're going too far. That was years ago. We decided based on the best medical information available."

"And how it's grown back. Look how the boils ceased."

Outraged, now: "How dare you lay that on me? Blame me for a system's injustice? We were who we were. I've taken care of you."

"How ironic. You actually believe you've been taking care of me. I'm not pausing another fifteen years to reclaim my body and my life."

"What does that mean? I won't let you do this, Irene. Not now. University is a nightmare. The Keynote Address in Lahore is coming up."

"You no longer let or don't let me do anything. Amputated, I've been mutilated."

No longer pretending to be doing homework, I stared, horrified. They'd passed caring who witnessed. My nightmare was coming true. Tonight my family will shatter. They are killing this family right now. Tonight. Stop this battle. Do not look away. My family.

My three words came out too late, too weak, slowly, inept. "Please," I pleaded. I begged. "Don't fight." No brothers to rescue me. I was alone to stop them. Of course, I'd blow it.

―

Their clash grew out of control, beyond any two miserable souls. They fought for control over plenty beyond control — us boys, each other, each others reactions. White hot, Mom embodied the pure, righteous seething rage of a generation of women who had reached their limits. In that moment, it didn't matter what she destroyed, Dad, the family, herself.

Poor Dad. He faced a choice deeply hidden and woefully obvious. Like a tragic character, he never saw the choice and could never make it. You didn't need to read Simone de Beauvoir or Virginia Woolf to see the choice, and he could quote both. Every day he and Irene stayed together, he faced a choice: either pay daily for the crimes of generations of men or grow. Accept her full agency, welcome the woman he loved into the same humanity he enjoyed. He never made the choice and never saw how sad his loss.

Instead, Dad set upon me. "We aren't fighting. It's a disagreement. You are old enough to appreciate the difference." Lip curled, trembling, he withdrew to his study. Poor, poor, tragic Dad. Coming home, expecting a safe port of call, he'd entered enemy waters with three rivals and one accuser. He must have been so lonely.

Later, Mom called me to her room; maybe she needed to explain or apologize or justify or merely talk. She slouched on the edge of her bed, her blue eyes cloudy. She tried to tell a witty story about the nurses proclaiming she could choose her new cup size, whatever she desired. But her voice lost its usual clever strength. "Emma always called me a washboard."

Then the confession: "I have four sons, not three. And the oldest and neediest demands so much, there's nothing left for you three. Nothing left."

Sure, or maybe you have one supreme son and three small make-believe husbands. I said goodnight. Nothing else to say.

## A place where anyone can hang out

I slunk back to my room, unable to escape my family in turmoil, the world in turmoil, both bent on destruction. The madness advanced ever closer, leaving little room to hide, confront, or flee.

One kid on a three-speed bicycle, riding to a place for anyone to hang out and nosh and cherish each other. An unmapped ancient manor with lots of rooms, up and down and behind hidden doors, and passageways to crawl spaces, or a bus crammed with singing people on an endless highway, or a cave with tunnels growing left, right, straight, up and down. I rode to the place in my head, staring at the ceiling, playing ceiling baseball, surrounded by books and maps. Little unopened bottles labelled Pfizer stood in a row on my shelf filled with ineffective syrup. Maybe someday I'd build the place outside in the real world too.

Until that magic day when I made my family whole and right, we remained five bags of unmet, unexpressed hopes and longings. We looked in vain to each other for fulfilment. Each of us found solitary obsessions and distractions to satisfy our cravings. Dad through his work; Pete, music; Stephen, sex and alcohol; Mom, her writing and stories. I resorted to books and imagination, searching for a way out. And food.

## Check out the freak, Thomas Starr King Junior High

It must have been a rough day, one where I took myself too seriously. My stomach probably hurt. A normal day. At lunch I wandered the grounds, snacking on a navel orange, and I popped. Not for the first time, my inner world shifted in an instant.

About ten guys huddled in a group eating lunch at two outdoor tables. My age, but they all wore sharply creased blue uniforms. Starched and stiff. Ten folded side caps. I'd never seen a mini-army inside junior high. I froze and stared. A couple of them noticed me. "Check out the freak."

A second one sneered, "Peacenik commie." Really. People said that, back then.

As I said, a normal, annoying day. Sure these characters pissed me off. Sure, I stood against my generation being militarized and programmed to hate. The entire bunch swivelled towards me with crossed arms, glaring eyes.

My larger-than-life, cosmic battle loomed. My blood raced, face hot, vision tunnelled. Sure, I'll defy ten large, uniformed dudes. I yelled. Stephen would have stepped in, cooled everyone down with a few words, stood up for me, and charmed these kids in uniform. Didn't happen. They'd kicked him out of school — nobody said why — so, he couldn't rescue me.

A couple of them launched in my direction. Nothing tentative in their steps. From across the commons, another uniformed figure approached the group. One shouted, "Sergeant!" Instantly all ten paused, leapt at tense attention. Straighter, stiffer, ten rigid hands hammered against ten brows in salute.

These students were not playing toy soldiers. No game, the guys were being trained for entry into a machine of destruction. Serious students in military uniforms saluted. Terrified and threatened, I burned with a fire of justice. I knew this fire well. Against some ancient offense, I flailed, clawing, screaming, and pounding. My enemy transcended these specific kids. In my mind the battle enlarged to cosmic proportions, my foes took on archetypal stature. My peripheral vision blurred; my universe narrowed, at the moment I pictured the battlefield widen.

In fact, archetypal forces seized me, not my schoolmate-soldiers. "Get out of Vietnam." With righteous fury, I threw my orange scraps in their direction.

## Instigating fights

"Mr. Robinson, I hoped to offer you an opportunity to tell your side of the story."

"Shouldn't my parents be here?"

"Oh, we can call them in for a formal hearing. But I'm sure you don't want to let it go that far. Let's see if we can settle this problem without causing you extra grief."

"Why was Stephen kicked out of school? The real reason? I heard Mrs. Thompson and Stephen were . . ."

"We took care of that problem. That's not why I summoned you. We want to avoid the same thing happening to you. Now, I asked a question. We received a report you hurled rocks at a group of students."

"I threw an orange. They razzed me. Called me a freak." Of course, I considered myself a freak. "Do you think I was looking to battle ten king-sized guys? Who are they?" Out the window to my left he had a view of a brick wall from another wing of the school. How many years, decades had he commanded the Boys' Vice Principal's Office with that view?

"You are new here, Mr. Robinson. I can't imagine what you're looking for. Those fine young men are part of the Junior ROTC, Reserve Officers Training Corps. Citizenship. Discipline." He didn't need to mention, qualities I lack. "King is an orderly school. We don't accept gangs here. We are going to keep it that way. Let's see if you can be cooperative."

"An orange, singular. Not rocks. I am not a gang." No gang would have me. Not the vatos or the surfers. Freaks are not in gangs.

"Other incidents, instigating fights. King isn't a fighting school." He shifted papers, glanced at them, shrugged. "You've only been here a few months and missed quite a bit of class; in fact, too much. Several of your teachers report you've been disruptive and you leave class without permission."

What would Stephen or Pete say? "I'm sick. Sometimes I need to go to the boys' room."

"If you are sick, we require a note from your parents. If you are sick as much as you've missed, we will need a letter from your Doctor."

"The doctors don't understand what's wrong with me."

"I don't either. Look, son, this could become serious. Fighting in school is serious, a police matter. Suspension, expulsion. We would be required to call in your parents, the authorities. Things you don't want."

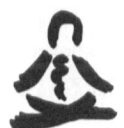

# The Asura, Inflammation Personified

### New school, 1968

BEFORE KING BOOTED ME out, I changed schools again. People said Bancroft Junior High better suited me, more academic. Bancroft demanded I enrol in a class there that King didn't offer.

Russian. Bancroft held a class in Russian. It could lead to a career path in one of the government intelligence services. Ironic, since that soldier boy called me a "commie peacenik." Most of my friends took French as their second language, but I ended up studying Russian through Junior and Senior High and into university. That's fine, I'll never use French.

Bancroft was too far to ride my bike. Getting there required over an hour on the bus and waking early. Off to a rough start, I skipped classes or showed up late.

Weary of being compared to Pete, the prodigy, I'd quit the piano. Hoping to expand my consciousness, I experimented with LSD and other hallucinogens. Meanwhile, my family continued its descent. Stephen's disappearances became longer. Mom also vanished several times for mysterious hospital stays. Some kind of breakdown. If the problem was hidradenitis suppurativa they would have said so. No, these were emotional. We didn't visit her in hospital. Who knows, maybe she wasn't even in hospital. Maybe she just needed to get away. Dad never explained her absences or returns, but his choked, accusatory tone directed blame at me. Without positive outlets for my anxieties and with no skills at inner growth, I boiled in a semi-constant state of misdirected rage.

Months would pass before I learned about the Asura. But, unless I found something inside worth fighting for, I threatened to become one, a destructive diminutive monster.

## The Realm of the Asura

The Asura are warlike, power-hungry mythological creatures from ancient India. They appear in the Vedas, texts that predate Buddhism by hundreds of years. The Asura fought with the gods for possession of amrita, a heavenly honey-like nectar of immortality. They yearn for power, and gleefully assault any foes, especially gods.

Passionate, the Asura burn for thrills and adventure. They can be easy to spot, often with smiles too wide, cars too fast, shiny jewellery, and shinier bedmates. An Asura makes a charming, fun-loving friend and breathtaking lover. With a pocket full of jangling quarters, they make the ideal buddies at a carnival or night on the town. They'll pour another pint for you at the pub or one more glass of Chardonnay and listen to your secrets.

To the Asuras, food, sex, and alcohol are tools. The Asuras don't care about those things, not really. Their sexual conquests aren't, in fact, about sex, their fortunes not about wealth, their wars not about land or gold. It's all about power and domination. The Asura crave control. They try to appear better, stronger, more clever than everyone. They pull strings and weave webs like spiders. As if endowed with six arms, they climb to the top of the towers of finance, the pyramids of authority, the heights of domination. As if three heads adorned them, they watch their backs and sides for usurpers and threats. They meet their comeuppance, of course. In their arrogance, they climb too high, piss off the wrong gods.

---

Once upon a time, one night, while most of the world slept, the Asuras gambled for it all, to go for broke, shoot the moon. Their six legs scrabbled up the towers' glass walls, seized the penthouse suite. Before this merciless onslaught, the security guards' defence crumbled. Humiliated, the night cleaners fled.

The three headed monsters tore open the liquor cabinet to ravage the oldest cognac, and snorted lines of cocaine on the pool table. They'd won it all, and they celebrated with a drunken rampage, smashing the flat screen TVs before passing out on the ripped leather upholstery.

The legitimate occupants seized the moment to punt the intoxicated, reckless kids out. The security guards with billy clubs cast the drunk Asuras out of the tower. They plummet to the ground dozens of floors below, fracturing their six arms, smashing their three faces.

Broken and smashed, but not dead. After all, nothing dies forever in myths and dreams and stories. Attempts to destroy hatred and contempt with violence can backfire. The legends say if you kill an Asura, and it spills as much as a drop of blood, a thousand more will demonically spawn from that single drop.

## Warring with gods

The ancient stories treat the Asura as real critters, living in their own corner of the world, with six arms and three faces, orange skin and spiky hair.

In Buddhism, the concept of the Asura evolved. The expression "asura" came to describe qualities within us all, symbolising the power-hungry, domineering side of regular folk. Inside each of us lurks a bellowing orange-red faced Asura, blazing with passion and fury.

The inner asura-state conceals the authentic self from others' eyes and especially from oneself. And our inner asura urges us to dismiss other's worth, to make oneself feel bigger by diminishing others. To eagerly brawl with any would-be challengers to our strength, savviness, or treasure.

After all, warring with gods demands full attention, with little space for introspection or empathy. If we're in the grip of the asura tendency, everyone and everything becomes tools for our battles or fools to be scorned or trashed. Far from being mindless drones of war, we scheme with intention. When reason and tactics fail, we seduce with cultivated charm.

> *Those in the world of the Asuras think of themselves as the most wonderful people. The energy of the world of anger is directed toward sustaining and enhancing this image. To ensure that others think of them in similarly glowing terms, they can never*

*reveal their true feelings but act in a fawning, obsequious manner....*
*Since their hearts are crooked, they can see neither themselves nor others correctly. Looking at things through the distorted lens of arrogance, they think they are larger than life. As a result, they neither desire to learn from others nor are they capable of honest self-reflection, both of which are the means to grow as human beings.*[25]
Daisaku Ikeda

The asura-state does not impede cognition, despite rising blood pressure and rolling heat in the belly. We can operate at a conscious level high enough to fake piety, wisdom, courage, and other virtues. High enough to simulate, as one scholar noted, a small "goodness of mind."[26]

I now know the flatterer longs to be sincere; the manipulator, to be trustworthy; the bully, to be genuinely courageous. The longing, no matter how faint, towards restoring our own dignity and recognizing that same dignity in others, holds hope. This is the hope of the contemptuous, warlike side of us all.

To appear right and decent, I envied and mimicked others' natural authenticity. In my heart, I knew my life could be much more. I, too, craved control, as my stomach, my family, and the world spun towards destruction. I now know — the monster inside was trying to protect me and to assert my poorly developed sense of self.

Too often I reacted aggressively, physically attacking or putting others down. But I was not an automaton. I'd been endowed with choices. I didn't want to hurt others; I wanted to stop hurting. To be brave, not angry. Instead of looking down on others, to just like myself.

Thus a crack in my arrogance formed; a sliver of the light of innate wisdom, kindness, and creativity dimly shone. In mom's dressing room hung a trifold mirror. While she was away, I put the three sides together around my head and looked at the reflections bouncing back and forth, as if they went on forever. At just the right angle, with my head tilted so, in a corner of the furthest mirror, I made out a crack, another reflection mirroring back, a hint of what might be.

I could look into that reflective shard and glimpse both an angry, frightened kid and a dignified, fierce warrior for justice. A hint of self-respect may have detoured my insatiable craving for validation. No longer a child, I had to discover my dignity and allow others theirs. I had to win this inner battle. Even I, an imploding, self-absorbed teen, might tentatively step toward my humanity and freedom, if I found the tools or someone with them.

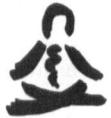

# Part of the World

### Diagnosis, Kaiser Permanente Hospital

LIKE A SOW BEAR and her cub, Mom and I propped ourselves across Doctor Goldberg's desk. We'd sat at other desks, across from other doctors, in other offices with degrees hanging on white walls.

"We now understand what is wrong with Keith." He addressed Mom. "The name is regional enteritis. It is an inflammation of the terminal ileum."

After years of hospitalizations, misdiagnoses, endless inconclusive tests, this might be the end of the pain. I hurt. The tests hurt. Being told my sickness was in my head hurt. Wondering if it was in my head hurt. Being exhausted all the time and not being able to do normal stuff hurt. Today might be the end of the hurt.

I didn't follow who he meant by "we" or what's a terminal ileum. Sounded final. But it's hopeful. He figured out what's wrong. He held my attention. Maybe today ends the pain, the endless shitting of undigested meals, not going outside in case a toilet wasn't available. A hopeful look plastered on my face. Please. Tell me I will be okay. Tell me the pain will end.

"It's rare," the doctor leaned back slightly, fingers steepled. They solved the puzzle. "Yours is my first case. A doctor named Crohn at Mount Sinai in New York first identified it. The cause is not clear. Currently, no treatments are available. Keith will probably require surgery at some stage. Meanwhile, we will track its progress." The disease's progress.

No treatment. They won't even try anything. Everything's the same. Still all alone. I'll never meet a girl, never play ball again. No good to anyone, never join the revolution. Be nothing.

Mom sat up, her arm raised protectively in front of me. The momma bear. She sounded the same as when she demanded answers from me. Who ate the cookies? Who didn't put away the dishes?

"What kind of surgery? What about diet? Do his nerves play a role? Should we send Keith to this Doctor Crohn?"

"We can watch it here. There isn't much more they can do in New York."

Mom's eyes narrowed. Protect her baby boy. "How bad can this become?"

"It probably isn't fatal, but he will have it his whole life. Most patients actually die from malnutrition. The diseased bowel grows unable to absorb nutrients." He glanced at chubby me. A doctor should notice I hurt. "Malnutrition isn't imminent."

Malnutrition, I understood. I am going to starve to death. Not imminent, but slowly.

Not permitted to chew my fingernails or scratch myself in public, I hid my hands in my lap under the edge of the metal desk. Using the nail of my right thumb, I knifed into the flesh under the second fingernail, then the third, until it hurt too much and on to the next. Once through all the fingers, I started again. My gaze swept the room for a wastebasket or other container if I puked.

Mom pressed. "And?"

"It's difficult to say, with few cases. Not to get ahead of ourselves, but at some point he may require a stoma."

"What's a stoma?" I queried, uncertain if I wanted the answer.

Before the doctor could reply, Mom answered. "A stoma is a bag, dear. It means they remove your bowels and you empty into a bag."

I wondered if a stoma would make the pain go away. I didn't ask.

We found the white-tiled men's room, then Mom's car.

Back home, Mom called us to the living room. Her voice, sombre and authoritative, left no crack for argument. Her petite frame towered over the same living room where she dragged the family to the edge, accusing Dad of wrongly causing her mastectomy, in the same home that my friends said visiting "hurts." Today, however, the room felt unfamiliar. Floaty.

I joined my family huddled in a circle. For once, we assembled with nobody having to first do this or finish that. For once, we didn't bicker about how people said this or that, the choice of words, in what order, or who was told what, when.

We stood enveloped in a white haze coming through the picture window over the LA basin. Not wanting to see their faces, my gaze drifted around the room, Mom and Dad's living room, as though for the first time. Her *New York Times* crossword puzzle lay open, near finished on a side table. Books and magazines lay scattered amongst furniture and Mom's house-plants. Mom and Dad's anecdotes and adventures lay behind each lamp, each decoration, picture, and hand-picked piece of furniture. Pleasing, sensible stuff, not expensive but memorable to one or both.

I hovered amongst their stuff, inside their memories. My feet carried me there, into this room I'd been a thousand times. Now I floated disconnected from the carpet or earth. Time paused and I paused, in a white frozen cube. My eyes wandered, unfocussed, in a room bathed in white. Not sure why nobody grabbed a seat.

Mom told everybody the news. Mom didn't smile. She smiled easily with friends, rarely with family. Her eyes, normally fragile wet forget-me-nots, became two unblinking sapphires. Mom took charge in righteous protector mode. Calm and focussed and fierce.

Dad paid careful attention, his neck at an awkward angle, didn't interrupt, and nodded. "Well, now we know. Now we know."

I plonked on the couch. And here, Dad, here you apologize for blaming me, declaring I made myself sick by eating fast. But I said nothing. For once, I shut up. Today was not about him.

Stephen stared at me, his face for once uncertain, eyebrows raised momentarily. He stepped in my direction, lifted a hand, then lowered it and spun back.

Pete talked about chanting ... transform your life.

I tried to put it together — what the doctor said and Mom reported. Finally, they named my plight — that's good.

I wasn't crazy — that's terrific.

Nothing to be done, rest of my life, surgery, starving to death — not great.

Sure, Pete, sure. Leave me alone; I'm not doing so well.

## Not my name

Stephen left the house as soon as Mom released us. Alone, I thought to curl up in bed. Instead, I paced in our room, from the closet to Stephen's unmade bed to the cat door and back. Use your noggin. Occasionally, walking made the bowel relax a bit. Or distract me. Clear out the white fog, figure this out. At that moment, my guts burned, a smoldering red fire in a fog. I couldn't concentrate. Concentrate. Work it out.

Giving my pain a name meant more than a hurray diagnostic victory. It's a promise. Goldberg's diagnosis promised that my disease exists amongst the recognized things. And I exist among the things of the world. Regional enteritis exists in the world, not imagination. Yes, the pain, the disease, and I were real. People become sick; our sicknesses come with names, and the possibility of treatment.

That's what the doctor meant by declaring, we understand what is wrong with you. Your malady has a name. My disease and I became part of human experience, part of the universe of named things. There's a book somewhere with a list of diseases and another book with a list of humans. Somewhere in the first book is regional enteritis and somewhere in the second is me. My disease exists, has a name. As do I.

My stomach blazed. I paced faster, kicked orphaned socks under my bed. Around and around the bedroom. Sure, but there's also the no treatment part, watching its progress while I starve, until I needed surgery or a bag. A bag of shit. Me, a pacing bag of shit. He said I won't die, but he didn't say how long I could live with it. Or how to live with my guts on fire, burning, not killing me, endlessly burning. Nobody taught how to handle school, pursue a career, or approach my crush, Evie. There's no way to try my best, no way to not quit.

Back and forth in the room, legs growing heavy, losing track of time. Once a year on TV, they showed those telethons for muscular dystrophy. They parade children, calling them "Jerry's kids," onto the stage in their wheelchairs. The little muscular dystrophy fighters. Not me. No little regional enteritis fighter here. My disease now had a name, but it wasn't my name. Now I will resist. I didn't know what I was, but, sure as shit, I will not be a little regional enteritis fighter.

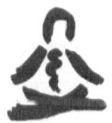

# "For those who work for peace."

## Hope, courage, confidence, North Hollywood

Pete took me to one of his meetings. Not what I expected. I anticipated going to a hall, with earnest white-haired spiritual types, as pale and wraithlike as the spirits conjured out of an ouija board. I expected a boring lecture. A Gandhi-esque Asian man in robes would spout incomprehensible eastern philosophy. Yeah, no, I got that wrong. Pete drove us to a private home in North Hollywood. We were late. People already jammed the living room, sitting on the carpet, clasping beads and reciting in unison out of small blue books.

Pete found a spot next to one guy. The guy directed his book towards Pete and pointed to the place they'd reached. Pete caught up to their chanting. I stayed in the back, without a little book or beads, unsure if they expected me to follow along. The chanting dragged on without a break or explanation. What were they reciting, in what language? They kept going.

I surveyed the packed room. The group faced a sizable black altar-cabinet-thing, an overgrown version of the small one hanging on Pete's wall. Mostly college aged and slightly older whites and a few Blacks and Latinos. Nobody my age. No Asians; no one resembled Gandhi. They looked like hippies, former hippies, and regular-looking folk.

After the chanting, they told their stories: overcoming drug problems, dropping out of school and returning, avoiding killing and being killed in Vietnam, reuniting with estranged families. None of it sounded spiritual or what I imagined as Buddhisty.

A woman named Joyce conducted the meeting sitting on the floor behind a little coffee table. Next to her sprawled a boy around six colouring while vying for the woman's attention. Crayons and colouring books surrounded him.

Joyce answered people's questions, her hands wide on the table or moving as she spoke. She engaged with each person, nodding with a slight smile. Without ignoring or brushing off the child, she stayed engaged with the participants.

The meeting seemed silly. I didn't have any of their problems. One guy, with a thin mustache and thinner western string tie, had a bunch of questions: "What does the chant mean? What are you chanting to? Is it a Buddha or an idol?"

Joyce leaned slightly towards the questioner; her eyes became owl-like orbs. "Nichiren Daishonin, a thirteenth century Japanese monk, started this Buddhism. He taught that chanting Nam-myoho-renge-kyo tapped our inner energy for transformation. We all have problems. How do we deal with our problems? Do we escape? Do we blame others?

"As Buddhists, we don't pray to the outside for answers," Joyce continued, elevating her chest and head. "Hope, courage, confidence are inside. Inside you, me, every one of us. It's inside. When you change, your circumstances change. Your life expands, the human revolution. It is the basis of lasting change, all other revolutions."

When she said, "It's inside," she jabbed her fingers towards her heart.

She reminded me of Nancy, the college student who'd come to our house. Joyce, older, shared with Nancy an ease, comfort, and powerful focus. Not gonna lie, a pulse-racing turn on. If Nancy and Joyce were typical of women in this group, I got why Pete joined. I looked around the room again for any young women near my age. No luck.

---

The participants demonstrated the same cheer as Nancy and the two men who came to the house, a sense of hope. I could not deny it — cheer I lacked. The world tore itself apart, my family tore itself apart, my stomach tore me apart. And these people stayed cheerful.

## Do not be driven from home

In my room, I was engrossed in James Baldwin's *Giovanni's Room*. It's the story of a young man named David who feels valued and seen solely by Giovanni. But Giovanni's room is a mess and too small for the both of them. He doesn't fit in the one place in the world where he experiences love. David suffers confusion about his identity, agonizes in guilt and shame, and feels lonely even with others.

Yup, my place hurt, a place of strife. I wished my family could be nurturing, protective, harmonious. Sure, we differed from others, but we weren't fundamentally flawed. We lived decent lives. Mom and Dad weren't criminals or hurtful. In fact, Mom and Dad's humanity, their consideration of the social consequences of their daily behaviour, I found pretty damn groovy. I admired them and found much to emulate. Nothing was wrong with us, but everything was.

Pete walked into my room. "What are you reading?"

"James Baldwin. Knock. What do you want?"

"Read *The Fire Next Time*. 'This is your home, my friend. Do not be driven from it; great men have done great things here.' It's all in there. Everything."

"Good memory. What do you want?"

"I have a rehearsal in Hollywood tomorrow and need your help setting up."

"Get Stephen. I'm sick." I hadn't seen Stephen all day. "Where's Stephen?"

"Gone. Father is searching for him. Look, I need this. This rehearsal is important. You're not so sick. I'll give you a ride somewhere. Where do you want to go?"

Stephen left home. Ran away. I should too. Head to Chicago. Join the revolution. "Wallichs Music City, since you are going to be in Hollywood. But it will cost you more than a ride. There's an album I want. Four dollars."

"What album?"

"Not your type. It's called the *Velvet Underground*. Andy Warhol made the cover."

"Be ready at one, little brother."

"We'll see how I'm feeling."

## A purple scarf, Venice Beach house

Pete tricked me. After the rehearsal, we had to tear down his equipment. We got his yellow Datsun pickup loaded with the electric pianos, amps, clavicle, cables. Then the drummer expected a hand and the sound guy too. The Hollywood heat and smog pressed down. *The Velvet Underground* and a ride cost too much sweat. Pete drove me to the record store. Then, "I need to run an errand."

"You only said the rehearsal." He duped me.

"It will be a minute. And there's somebody I want you to meet."

---

He drove us out to Venice Beach, with me fidgeting in the small truck's cab. Forty minutes at least there, forty minutes home. Not a minute. Pissed me off. My fingers traced the album's edges through the paper bag on my lap as I grew angrier by the minute. Every step on the brakes grated; every shift of gears jerked. My new album waited. Stupid me, caught in his trap.

Under other circumstances, Venice would be cool, with skaters and surfers and artists, live music, definitely girls on the boardwalk. But not today and not with Pete, running his "errand." Today I am a fly in his web and am going to resist.

He pulled up to a peach coloured bungalow. The heat building up in the cab could warp and ruin the album before I ever heard it. So, I left the window open a crack and stashed *The Velvet Underground* under the truck's seat.

I dragged myself out of the truck, squinting in the blazing sun. The smog lightened near the beach; my mood darkened. Two older men talked enthusiastically on the porch, arms loose, leaning towards each other. One sported a handlebar mustache under a floppy hat. The other wore a tight Afro and toothy smile. They said hello as we stepped up the stairs. Pete said hello, didn't introduce me, and inquired if "Larry" was still there. Afro guy said, "He is leaving soon." Mustache guy tilted his hat brim and smiled at me. They gave off the same vibe as the people at the North Hollywood gathering. Something about their type. These people and their smiles irritated me. Didn't they realize there's a war?

---

Inside, we took off our shoes. In the hall and living room, more Buddhist types gabbed in clusters of three or four. Full throated laughter punctuated their animated conversations. Of course, they weren't laughing at me, but still, I didn't get the joke. Against the far wall of the living room rose another black altar-cabinet-thing, similar to the one at the gathering in North Hollywood. It seems to occupy the entire wall. In front of the altar stood a shiny black lacquered table with two unlit candles on either side.

Five or six people, mostly women of different ages, gathered around one tall guy. "This is who I want you to meet," Pete said. We joined the little circle. Tall guy was adorned with huge ears and a generous sprinkling of freckles. The ring of devotees listened breathlessly.

I had a hard time following the speaker's monologue, laced with strange foreign terms. A few words popped out. Surf the waves, don't drown in them, fulfil your promise, develop your life, realize your potential. He spoke with intensity and confidence. Cool surfer.

Me, not cool. Antsy and irritated, my eyes wandered, the heat in my guts spreading. Pete set me up. The fires merged: my inflamed stomach, my anger at Pete's manipulation, the vice-principal's pressure, our family in flames, napalm, assassinations and riots in the streets. Burning alone in a peachy house in Venice and surrounded by strangers who didn't dig it and are smiling.

I surveyed the room, not seeking a friendly face. My misery sought company. All these faces appeared friendly, encouraging and nodding to each other. I scanned the room for the lady who came to our house, Nancy. Maybe a friend of hers is here. But it would have been so lame to ask.

Tall surfer guy wrapped things up. "Actually, I'm late for a meeting in Santa Monica." He wheeled, kneeled in front of the altar. One hand held beads. With a gong in the other hand, he struck a bell by the black table. It's a cue. They knelt and chanted three times slowly in unison. Despite my determination to be miserable, I found the slow harmonious chant magnetic.

They stood. Pete intercepted the guy on the way to the door. In one breath, "Larry, this is my little brother. I'm really concerned about him. He's thinking of running away from home. He isn't healthy; it's serious, a serious stomach disease." Pete's voice strained. And tears. Pete's eyes filled with tears.

I didn't understand. Pete knew I wanted to run away? I never said anything. Those were tears. He was crying. Big brother worried about me, *really concerned*. He cares about me. I am pissed, and he wept.

Larry caught my eye, glanced at Pete. Then, he focussed back on me with a small smile and a crinkle of his freckled nose. The slightest tilt of his head. I readied for an argument, the epic debate, my finger on a primal trigger. Watch my righteous protest against superstitious religion, the opiate of the masses.

"Practising puts you through changes, stirs up the dirt." His bright eyes focussed on me, but gentler than the cool surfer I imagined moments before. "Blaming others doesn't help. Blaming society doesn't make anything better. People built society. We can rebuild it to serve people." He leaned to Pete, who wiped his eyes. "I don't have much time. I'm already late." He started towards the shoes by the door. Halted. Reversed, lingering. No rush.

"Here, I have something for you." Facing me, Larry reached into his jacket pocket, pulled out a purple scarf. Lovely. He neatly rolled his prayer beads in the scarf, then handed the burrito-like package to me. "These are for young people who work for peace. We can talk again."

Back in the pickup, I held the compact purple package, confused about what just happened. I can't use his beads. Surfer Larry will need them, not me. I returned to being a kid again, not angry anymore, a miserable kid. Pete didn't so much as tell the surfer my name. I wasn't anyone. A pathetic kid, a wise-ass. Yet Larry saw me, talked to me as an adult, a person.

## Philosophical Research Society, Reading Room

I endeavoured to learn about Buddhism on my own. Figure this out for myself. A library near our house held lots of books on philosophy, including Buddhism. I escaped there. Most of what I read confused me, dry and opaque. Through the thick, dry, impossible reading, one idea struck me. They described the Buddha as observant, fully engaged, yet unattached. Far out. To wander the lands by foot or bus, possibly by plane, committed, involved, yet never bound, pulling small levers of peace and freedom.

Back home, lying on my back on the bed, *The Velvet Underground* on the turntable, Nico singing "I'll Be Your Mirror." A Nico or a Nancy might wander with me. Figure out what I can do; move towards the peace I craved.

My family remained my family. My guts remained my guts. Incurable. Untreatable. Not much I could do about either. One choice remained: change myself.

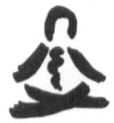

# In the Middle of Something

June 5, 1968
Dear Sister Carmelita,
I am writing from home because I didn't go to school today. Was up very late ~~last night~~ and my stomach bothered me all night. I miss piano lessons, but mostly miss talking to you. I didn't know who else to ask. Actually, I don't know what to ask. I just wanted to write you.
Last night I went to the headquarters for the McCarthy for President campaign. I came home around 10:30. McCarthy was behind, but I still thought he ~~might would~~ might win. Then when I got home I went to bed. Dad woke me in the middle of the night to tell me the news. The radio says they don't know yet if Kennedy ~~is going to die~~ will survive.
Another Kennedy shot. How can it be?
You always paid attention to me. I'm in the middle of something. Most of the time I am outside but this time it is like everything is going on around me. All these events happening around us, and we are part of them, but I don't feel anything. I should understand it, but I don't.

Maybe I should be shocked, but I'm not. Or I
don't know how to be shocked. I don't know
how to feel about what is going on, other
than I am angry. But I don't know what to do
with anger anymore.
They killed Malcolm X and what, two months
ago, killed Martin Luther King and now
this. And I thought, oh well, but I shouldn't
think that, I should have other thoughts,
more deep. We just watch. We are the ~~news~~ new
watchers. We are the news and we are
watching the news but we aren't really part
of it. But it is going to ambush us. That's
for sure. What does it mean that
assassination is the new reality. Not old
enough to remember the old reality. It is
~~like a crossroads~~ an intersection of ~~family
politics and news events~~ my family and the
news. They are coming together and I don't
know what it means. To me. To anyone.
My brother Pete says we should chant for
peace. Maybe he is right. I am considering
trying it. It is a funny thing to ask you but
you are the only person who understands
about prayer and faith. What do you think?
Keith

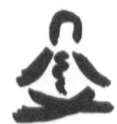

# "I trust you, Yo-chan."

## Yoshiko's story

DADDY'S NAME WAS TOKUZO Yamamoto. He named me Yoshie Yamamoto, but someone at the town hall messed up and entered Yoshiko on my birth certificate. To this day, villagers call me Yo-chan. Now I am Yoshiko Robinson.

You would have liked my dad, a rebel and a creative type. Dad loved to sing and drink. He painted water-colours, drew and wrote stories in *sumi* ink — an artist-farmer. Men of his generation called their wives "wife" or "mother," or "*oi*" (hey). Dad was different. He called Mom by her name, Emiko. For me, my brother and sister, with the day winding down, tucked into our futons, he'd tell us folktales and sing lullabies.

## Room to move, Yellow Sea

Mom and Dad suffered from war. They married in Manchukuo, the quasi-nation in Manchuria the Japanese built and ruled. In his restless youth, he left Tottori Prefecture for art school in Tokyo. Art freed his mind, but crowded Tokyo cramped him. He craved seeing the wide world of space and possibility.

At first, Dad avoided conscription — too short for the Imperial Navy — but didn't avoid the sea. In the thirties, he cooked on freighters up and down the coast of Asia. They made port in Pusan, Shanghai, Hong Kong. They hauled the raw materials and finished goods to build the Japanese Empire, an empire sailing to destruction.

Life on board meant cramped quarters, brutal hours, merciless lines of command and discipline. The cook slung dozens of meals from a scorching galley the size of a closet. Coming from the open Tottori countryside, Dad's body longed for room to move; his mind, for freedom.

Dad drew pictures of his mates and sang for them. The cook holds a privileged position on any ship at sea. Outside of the galley, his mates and the officers treated him well and granted him latitude impossible for a deckhand. After all, everyone on board, from bridge officers to the lowest engine room grease monkey, wants a little extra fish in their soup.

Typical of sailors, military or merchant, Dad drank hard, but with saké, his size proved a weakness. Too quickly and too often, the saké drank him.

## Dreams of the open roads, South China Sea

Late one warm summer night, after the captain and officers finished watch, they relaxed on deck. Dad sang traditional folk songs like "Sendou Kouta," The Ferryman's Song[27]:

> *You and I are withered pampas grass,*
> *By the riverside*
> *You and I will never blossom*
> *Only pampas grass*
>
> *You and I may live or die,*
> *The river flows just the same,*
> *The moon reflects off pampas grass*
> *So let's live on, ferrymen on the river*

The officers listened, put the playing cards away, their cups in hand. For a few minutes, these world-hardened sailors became little boys again, wrapped in Dad's clear, echoing voice.

The officers headed below, bellies and hearts full. Dad stayed above, enjoying the night sea air. A little time alone to ponder his future, breathing free air and trekking open roads. Start a new life, maybe find a wife.

But first, continue art studies. He'd submitted his cook's resignation papers. Once they made port in Hong Kong, he'd attend classes in Chinese painting. If things got worse and war broke out, hop another freighter back up to Dalian, the port dubbed "Gateway to Manchuria," catch the train to Hsinking. Locate land to homestead, paint landscapes, learn Manchurian folk songs. Manchukuo was a big land, open and hidden from the troubles of the world. Dad harboured a plan.

## Lies and reality, Hsinking, Manchukuo

Mom worked for families of the officers of the Imperial Kwantung Army, Japanese forces in charge of Manchuria. The Kwantung, elite troops of the Empire, answered to no one, often not Tokyo, and certainly not the puppet Manchu government. Mom served their families and household needs. They paid her well, much better than back home. And they paid in solid yen, not the depreciating Manchukuo yuan. Mom could remit to her family in Tottori.

Mom volunteered to journey to Manchuria. Like millions of young Japanese, she'd been recruited to become a colonist in Manchukuo. An intense propaganda campaign convinced her to aid in building a new modern society. Asian values would create harmony between Japanese, Korean, Chinese, Mongols, and Manchurians. "With the support of Japan, China, and Manchukuo, the world can be in peace."

The propaganda turned out to be lies. The Japanese rulers starved and enslaved the locals. They confiscated the Manchurian lands and conducted live human bio-warfare experimentation. Naked Manchurian and Mongol beggars packed the streets of Hsingking, the capital. Those horrors lay in the future or remained hidden.

In late 1940, the South Manchukuo Railway brought Tokuzo Yamamoto to Hsinking. An acquaintance told him about a girl from the same region in Tottori.

Her name was Emiko. They married in Manchukuo, and in August 1944 she became pregnant with my eldest brother. One year later, their lives crumbled.

We keep an old black-and-white photo of Mom from those days. Every time we dig it out, Keith comments on how much she resembled me, "intelligent, caring, striking." I examine that photo and consider her feelings for Dad and her hopes, the lies she heard and torments she endured. Makes me warm and enraged and determined.

In the picture, Mom was around eighteen or nineteen. Ahead lay unimaginable suffering. Ripped apart from Dad, Mom became a refugee, abandoned by her own country to trek across Asia on foot. Her first child starved to death in her arms. Yet, she survived, built a harmonious family of purpose and joy. Because of all she endured, I am determined to create a better future for those I can.

## The war ends but their horror begins

On August 8, 1945, two days after Hiroshima, the Soviet Union declared war on Japan. Stalin's Red Army and the Mongolian People's Army invaded Manchuria at midnight, August 9. Over 1.5 million troops with 55 hundred tanks swept into Manchuria from three sides. The Manchu Army either surrendered to the Soviets or mutinied against their Japanese masters.

Around two million Japanese colonists lived scattered throughout Manchuria. The Japanese military ordered women, children, and the infirm to evacuate at once with what they could carry.

They conscripted every boy and man, including Dad, to defend the Empire. Size, age, and health no longer mattered. All became fodder for a machine of destruction. Regular people paid dearly for the atrocities of militarism.

World War II ended after a couple of weeks with the Japanese surrender. Tokuzo and Emiko's suffering began. The Soviets seized Dad and hundreds of thousands of Japanese soldiers and civilians.[28] Dad became one of millions of Stalin's slaves, sent to Siberian forced labour camps.[29]

Mom carried my four-month-old brother east by foot across Manchuria. They joined a group of several hundred women, children, and elderly refugees.

At first, a unit of the Japanese Army accompanied them, ten soldiers. That didn't last. Somewhere in the Changbai Mountains, the soldiers told the group: "You're holding us back. Your kids are too slow and your babies wail. The Russians will hear. We're cutting you loose."

That night, they camped under the trees. The next morning, the soldiers had disappeared. The group huddled. "Certainly we are alone. We must make it to safety, no matter what. We must survive." The women and children continued alone, but united, determined. Later that day, they found the bodies of the ten Japanese soldiers, stripped of weapons.

She reached Pusan, Korea, against all odds. The baby didn't. Along the way, she stopped producing milk; my brother died. The US Navy took her from Pusan back to Kyushu, Japan. She stayed at Dad's parents' house waiting for him to return.

And waited. After three and a half years, a US ship carried him from Vladivostok to a repatriation centre at Maizuru port in Kyoto. Dad had survived Siberia.

At Maizuru, a doctor examined him. They inoculated him for cholera and typhoid and sprayed him with DDT. They exchanged his Soviet-issued winter clothes for civilian clothing. Volunteers fed him steamed sweet potatoes and tea.

Once she got him home, she removed the donated clothes. He'd shrunk, cheeks sunken, no meat, skin hanging limply off his skeleton. An oval scar marked his left side. The scar looked clean. Mom didn't ask about it. Questions could wait. Her husband came back from hell to her; that's all that mattered. She lowered him into the steaming bath. They had all the time in the world.

## The indigo fields, 1950

Over six million Japanese nationals remained in China and other Asian countries. The Japanese government and the US occupation forces needed to repatriate and settle them. Air raids had levelled Tokyo and other cities. The government opened uninhabited lands for settlement — swamps, mountain tops, remote islands, sand dunes.

Dad found out about a village called Aino, meaning the indigo fields, on an isolated side of Daisen mountain. What could they grow there? No-one knew. Aino was not completely uninhabited. Wild boar, foxes, and ferrets lived there forever without the intention of sharing the land easily.

In Aino, Mom and Dad were blessed with another son, Yusaku. He grew up to be intelligent, endlessly curious, with a dry wit. Unlike Dad, he grew tall, broad shouldered, and solid. And, unlike Dad, my elder brother holds his liquor. We weren't close growing up. But now we've grown into the dearest of siblings and friends, travelling together and assembling these family memories.

---

About a year later, 1951, Josei Toda became Soka Gakkai's second president. They had around three thousand members. Toda-sensei made a monumental determination — to convert 750 thousand households before his passing. Over the following six years, until his death, Toda's humanistic philosophy spread to every corner of Japan. His hopeful message reached our blink-and-you'll-miss-it hamlet. Aino hides in the most isolated south-west corner of Honshu Island, Tottori Prefecture. Daddy joined Soka Gakkai around 1956. I was three years old.

The Japanese government and society mistreated those who returned from the Soviet camps. Post-war Japanese society suspected them of being Communist agents. Their communities made it hard for them to get back on their feet and excluded them from jobs, education, housing, and basic health care.

They survived Stalin's death camps but their maltreatment continued. Many of the men lived the rest of their traumatic lives in shame, hiding their past, even from their families.

Dad was different. After joining Soka Gakkai, he lived with self-respect and gratitude. He appreciated surviving Stalin's camps, and appreciated Mom and their life in Aino village. He even missed the sawdust enriched black Russian bread of the camps.

Although we were poor dirt farmers, Dad had pride. He listened to others attentively, as talented singers do. I am so glad that when Soka humanism reached his ears, he heard.

But Dad didn't merely listen. At the important times, he spoke up for justice, including to elders. He argued with the local priests, the village chief, with anyone who tried to knock us down.

One time, a high-ranking priest in a nearby temple badmouthed Soka Gakkai. He claimed new religions insulted ancestors and violated the venerable traditions of the area. Dad heard that the priest hinted of hells awaiting Soka adherents in his sermons. "It's risky to become associated with these dangerous groups."

Well, Dad planned to engage in an old-fashioned debate. Everyone, even the local Soka Gakkai leaders, told him to leave it alone. Dad couldn't. He rode his horse Dannoko down to that temple armed with righteous determination. He told the priest how much his life had gained from practising with Soka Gakkai.

"I've learned to trust in myself, not promises from the mighty. I've learned to create hope and how to be free. Don't preach to me about hell. I've been to hell, spent three and a half years in labour camps across Siberia, while you lounged here in comfort. You can't scare me with superstition. New religions are dangerous, you preach? How much good did your old religions do for our country?"

---

Why did Dad argue so quickly? At first, it embarrassed me. As I grew older, I recognized he defended us quickly. Once my younger sister, Chie, and I assisted in the field. Well, that day we weren't helping; we were munching ripe mulberries off the bush. Mom and Dad planted mulberry bushes for the leaves, not the fruit. Mom and Yusaku collected the leaves to feed her silkworm larvae on her sericulture trays. Chie and I enjoyed the fruit.

Anyway, that day, the man from the Agriculture Co-operative was talking to Dad. Going on about what Dad should plant or subsidies for chemicals or some such. I didn't follow what he talked about, but I recognized the know-it-all tone. The expert spoke down to the hick.

"Turn downhill," Dad said. "Look through those bushes. All the way. What do you see?"

"What? Yonago Bay?"

"That's right, the Japan Sea. Storms head right here. We are four hundred metres up. Come back in January when the snow covers three metres thick, high as the eaves, snapping branches. Don't be forcing crops on us that won't last through our winter. We Aino village people are poor, but we aren't ignorant peasants. We have educators and graduates farming here. No different than everyone, we are struggling to survive."

Chie and I listened with pride. "See, elder sister, we enjoy delicious food. We sleep in warm futons. Our school uniforms may not be new, but our clothes are clean."

Our eyes met. "Yes, our family is warm and harmonious, thanks to Mommy and Daddy's efforts. They grow our food fresh in the summer and fall and preserve it for the winter. Some families borrow money from gangsters to survive the winter."

## Slaughtering a cow, Autumn, 1960

Dad said a cattle market and slaughterhouse are no place for women or kids. Feed and raise our dear cows for months to watch them drop dead with one electric shock to their beautiful heads. That settled it, no beef for me. When they took the farmers and agents to the slaughterhouse killing floor, only Dad stayed to watch his animals die.

One time, he sold a cow at the market, then headed straight for the nearest drink shop. He drank his fill, then stumbled out, vomiting, losing his dentures. Before passing out, he climbed into the back of the cart hitched to our brown mare. His baby, Dannoko, knew the way home. The white diamond patch on her forehead led the way. Nobody knows if she halted at the Habuki railway crossing and every red light. She got him home.

"You carried him home again." My brother, Yusaku, praised her, stroking her flanks. "What a good girl." She appeared proud, swishing her tail and snorting, her brown eyes wet.

Dad slunk into the house, a shamed sailor's footstep, sliding his feet over the tatami. "I hate that rubbing sound," Mom complained, as she stabled Dannoko.

The next day, to make amends with Mom, he rose before dawn, fetched the small stool and bucket to milk the remaining cows. I also woke early and asked, "Tell me where you went, Daddy? I will search for your dentures." He forgot and besides, he made himself too busy to answer or make eye contact with me, his head down, squeezing out the hot, rich milk.

"Don't marry a sailor," Mom said in that fed-up tone of every mother since the invention of ships and booze. At least that time we didn't receive a call to fetch him from the local police station.

## Three crows, 1962

Yes, we were poor. I didn't grow up with toys. Don't feel sorry for me. I enjoyed the happiest wild childhood, not bored for a minute, with mud on my face and my knees always scraped. Our family accumulated our kind of wealth. A playground of lush, dynamic nature surrounded us. I frolicked in bushes and fields, played with animals, climbed and fell out of trees plucking persimmons and figs.

Two village girls and I were inseparable friends. We became known as the three crows of Aino. We raced each other the four kilometres downhill to elementary school, usually late. Coming home, if the weather was good, took much longer with so many fascinating distractions. Tramping around in the bushes, looking for a place to pee, foraging our after-school snack. I gathered bamboo leaves for Dannoko and the cows' snack.

In the spring I ate river parsley and sorrel. I foraged wild Asiatic lilies to share with the family. Exploring and rummaging for everything was the most fun. Playing in the creek, I forgot everything they taught us in school. In the summer, I ate edible flowers, wild blueberries and raspberries, and tiny tart crabapples. In the fall, chestnuts and sweet persimmons. I proudly presented to Mom the edible mushrooms I found on the way home from school.

---

One fall day after the sweet yam harvest, us three crows flew a shortcut across a farmer's field. This farmer started a bonfire of the field's stubble and straw. Our sharp eyes found yam tubers left behind. We were thrilled to gobble them raw, but the fire was too tempting.

So the three of us, eight to ten-years-old, had an after-school barbeque. The farmer spotted us ragamuffins from up the mountain. "Koraa! You rascals get off my land." We dropped the yams and took flight towards Aino.

I didn't go home. I went with the middle crow, Harumi, one year older than me. Her family was somewhat more affluent than us Yamamotos. They let me take a bath in their luxurious tub and fed me dinner. Harumi's little sister, Pauline, tried to play with us big girls. After dark, their mother sent me home.

Mom was pissed off. "Where have you been? Why did you even come home? Just stay there and eat their food and join their family."

Was she kicking me out? I was in big trouble. I gathered Chie. "We have to leave home, little sister."

We went to the other side of our field under an evergreen tree. "Tonight, Chie, we will sleep here. Tomorrow, somewhere."

It was dark, but Yusaku knew where I'd go. He came and dragged us home. "Mom said you girls can come home. Don't ever make me do this again."

## Latitude and generosity

Our house's front entry gathered neighbours, distant relatives, and bill collectors. People leaned or squatted, too polite to come all the way inside. They gossiped, sought tips on foraging mountain fungi and vegetables, or asked for marital advice. Mom sent them home with a jar of her miso paste, or her soy sauce, tofu, or fermented vegetables. The kids who ate store-bought were so lucky. Why couldn't I enjoy refined white rice or processed, bottled soy sauce? But now I appreciate that I ate the best — Mom's.

Decades later, in 1993, Ikeda-sensei came to Vancouver. He gave a talk on living life joyfully and said that we would find true wealth by having latitude and generosity. Make room for others, a place at the table, or a cup of tea. When I heard those words, I realized how richly my family lived.

## On the farm, 1953–1963

Nineteen families settled in tiny Aino village. Too small for maps, don't bother looking it up. The families worked together, clearing land, erecting shelters, planting and harvesting. The saying went, even the cats lent a paw. Our two tabbies, Tanuki and Kitsune, kept the rats from our meagre stores.

Dad built our house at the top of the village, a single log at a time. Dad added to our home over the years, gradually adding stalls for ten cows and Dannoko's stable. He also built a shed for pickling kim-chee, daikon, green striped melon, and the mountain vegetables and fungi Mom foraged.

In the beginning, no one knew what to grow. Mr. Kato planted bamboo. This proved handy for the entire village. We used bamboo for many things around the farm — stakes for vegetables, poles, laths in construction, and fences. And, in the spring, the baby shoots are delicious and nutritious if the wild boar didn't devour them first.

Every evening, I lit the wood fire to heat everybody's bath. Most times, I screamed, opening the door to the hall on my way to the wood stack. Dead chickens, ducks, goats, hung from hooks, blocked my way. Dad aged them after slaughter, draining the blood from their necks into buckets. Dead hanging animals and buckets of blood decided for me: no chicken, duck, beef, or goat meat on my plate.

Once when I was eight, Mom braised mackerel in soy sauce. She plucked the oily, smelly fish out of the pot with chopsticks. The same chopsticks ended up at my dinner place. I touched them to my lips and gagged. No fish for me — the texture, the smell, the fishiness.

Mom and Dad tried growing anything — cabbage, watermelon, sugar beets, silkworms, daikon. No matter what we grew, we never got the best price. Our produce ripened late on the mountain compared to more fertile areas. Then, we needed to transport our product to market. The closest city, Yonago, lay twenty kilometres down rough mountain roads. Our veggies always received low prices.

## Watermelons to Hiroshima, 1963

To fetch better prices, Dad thought of hauling their produce to market on the Pacific Ocean side, in Hiroshima. But nobody in Aino owned a truck. Dad found a guy in a neighbouring village willing to rent and drive his flatbed. They made a perfect pair: Dad didn't drive; the guy with the truck didn't drink.

Yusaku joined the expedition. At thirteen, my elder brother, built wide as a barn door, stood taller and toiled harder than most adults.

In Junior High, bullies went after the small, pretty boys. The victims adopted Yusaku as their protector. One time Mom told us to pick up flour on our way home from school. He didn't like his little sister hanging around. "Don't come close to me. I don't want my mates to see me with you." He easily manhandled the ten kilo bag. Going home, we lingered at the bus stop. He sat on the bench, the sack of flour in his lap. I stood aside, keeping a proper distance. In an instant, two smaller boys from his class sat on either side, gorilla children guarded by the great Silverback.

Taking watermelons to Hiroshima, Dad knew the big city market dealers and smarties would try to rip off little country folk. Dad trusted Yusaku's reliability and good sense. Since 1970, the drive to Hiroshima takes three hours over the smooth 100 km/hr toll Chugoku Expressway. But in those days, it took all night over rough mountain roads to reach the market for the 5 a.m. opening. Of course, Dad sang to pass the time as they bumped along.

We wrapped each watermelon in rice straw blankets to survive the bumps. I wiped the melons clean, attached the confident "Daisen Watermelon" sticker, and assisted loading. If the melons, raised on rich volcanic soil, arrived intact, they'd fetch strong prices.

The plan succeeded. That first trip, Dad made 50,000 yen, which was around sixteen hundred US dollars in today's buying power. An astounding haul in 1963. And he didn't drink it. The cash came home to Mom. They were elated.

The next weekend, they tried again. This time, after paying for the truck and the driver and gas, they brought home less. They drove to Hiroshima one final time. Not worth it. Yusaku wasn't sleeping the entire weekend, ruining his school. If they kept it up, eventually they'd meet an accident. And melon season neared its end.

## Red Dragonfly, 1963

Two farms down the mountain from us lived the unfortunate Kato family. The Katos hoped for children. She miscarried or delivered stillbirths two or three times. Then they had a son.

One afternoon, Mom said, "Yo-chan, stop playing. Go help Kato-san." I scrambled down to their house. With mud on my face, my soup bowl haircut, I was not a cute Japanese doll.

Mrs. Kato met me at their house's entrance, dressed for the field. She wore *monpe* pants with strings tying the legs; a sweaty bandana screened her head and neck. The baby lay by her in a wicker basket.

"Turn around."

She wrapped a long scarf around me, making a sling on my back. She spun me again to bind me in the front. Bent down, her enormous buck teeth blocked my view. She'd fashioned a *noraboshi* hood out of the thin cotton bandana to protect her face from the sun. Still, she looked older than Mom, her skin stretched and shrivelled like a dried persimmon.

She gathered the baby and placed him in the sling. Around four months old, he didn't squirm, cry, or resist. Pink blotches pocked his chalky skin. Why isn't he crying, *ogyaa-ogyaa*?

"I'm off to the field." And she disappeared.

---

The sling wrapped him to my back. While waiting, I sang a song that Dad taught me, "Akatonbo," Red Dragonfly. I barely felt his weight. Singing on the path in front of their home, the heat of the silent, motionless baby boy warmed my teeny back. I can't remember his name. The mandarin orange sun descended through the western sky.

> *Red dragonflies in the sunset*
> *When was it that I watched them on someone's back?*
> *In mountain fields*
> *we gathered mulberries*
> *In small baskets*
> *Or was it just a dream?*
> *A red dragonfly in the sunset*
> *On the tip of a bamboo pole*[30]

The next morning, while I ate breakfast, Mom chopped vegetables at the sink. Mom's back faced me as she worked. "Kato-san's baby died." Chop, chop.

I never forgot. I'd turned ten or eleven, my grandson's age now. The baby on my back, sick but alive, warm. Yesterday he lived and now he is dead. Where did his life go?

Over time, Mrs. Kato successfully birthed two healthy girls. Now and then, I baby-sat them or Mom would send me to their house with cabbages or her homemade soy sauce. If Mrs. Kato didn't answer the door, I'd find her in their farm shed. She'd be squatting on the dirt floor in a corner, surrounded by dirty tools and dust, smoking. Staring.

The Katos did not suffer endlessly. The older daughter, once of age, joined Soka Gakkai. She left Aino village to pursue a nursing career, then returned home, bringing a touch of joy to the ill-fated family.

## War movies

One day in the fourth grade, the entire school gathered in the gymnasium to watch a dramatically narrated movie. Stirring music and grainy footage told the patriotic stories of brave kamikaze pilots and their noble sacrifice.

After school, I told Mom. This time, she stared right at me. Her eyes were clear, but her voice shook. "There's nothing noble about war. Nobody wins. People always suffer. War brings out the worst in people. When we were leaving Manchuria, the Russian soldiers came. Which one would steal our food? Which one would rape? Some were kind. Yo-chan, listen: there is no good from war."

## The Way of Tea

Mom and Dad barely afforded our school fees, so music or dance classes remained out of reach. In fact, Yusaku never attended high school. But Dad intended to educate me about the world and culture. One day, he took me to an elderly lady's house. She taught the Way of Tea and built a proper tea house for classes. She showed the tea house to Dad and me. Its low entrance forced all who entered, noble or common, to bow.

Dad could not pay for her regular classes. To pay, he repaired an appliance for her, or bartered a sack of mountain vegetables. She taught us the ritual, how to handle the utensils, at her kitchen counter, not the tea house. More than the ceremony, we learned respect for all life, respect for each other, gratitude, and culture.

Later, in high school, I caddied at a golf course in the summer. In the winter, I worked at a mountain inn, doing light housekeeping and as a kitchen assistant. During dinner service, I prepared side plates and ran dishes. I frustrated the staff with my rough manner. They'd sneer, "Farmer's daughter plops food in the bowl like pig slop."

The mistress said, "C'mon, handle the delicacies with class."

One time, two university students on a ski holiday stayed at the inn, rich kids, full of themselves. Barely a couple of years older than me, but they acted as though they owned the mountain.

The kitchen sent out a sashimi course. At the prep table lay two sauces in identical dispensers — soy and Worcestershire. I grabbed the Worcestershire by mistake and took it out with the fish. One kid screamed bloody murder.

The mistress came and gave me shit and ordered me to apologize and bow extra low, head on the tatami low. I learned a few new words that evening.

Despite my clumsy farmer's ways, my skill at the tea ceremony surprised the mistress. "Hmm, country girl does grasp a thing or two."

I enjoyed that job. Meals, a daily hot bath, clean sheets to sleep on, and they paid me. When High School began in April, Mom and Dad paid for my uniform. The money I made at the inn covered my school supplies, fees, room, and meals.

## Unlimited dreams, 1964

Despite the horrors they'd seen and all the hardships they had been through, Mom and Dad still had hope and supported Soka Gakkai's efforts for peace. One evening, the summer after the death of the Kato's baby, our family strolled together to a Soka Gakkai discussion meeting. On a rare family outing, Mom, Dad, me, my brother Yusaku, and little sister, Chie, marched to the next village down the mountain.

How times changed. Some years ago, Aino Village disappeared from maps altogether as an older neighbouring village annexed it. Nowadays the area has golf courses and resorts and bed-and-breakfasts, a micro-brew pub, farmers' market. An organic hipster bakery now stands at the village foot.

How hipster? They always seem to be closed or sold out when Keith and I visit, hungering for quality bread.

Back in '64, around twenty members met that evening at one family's home. Before the meeting, the hosting family rambled door-to-door, explaining to the neighbours we'd be gathering, hoping we don't disturb them. Some of the old-fashioned neighbours didn't appreciate Soka Gakkai.

Country folk gathered for the meeting — kids and grannies and farmers fretted about weather and crops. We caught up on news (and local gossip), whose daughter was expecting, whose son left for agriculture school. The adults talked about faith and daily struggles and modest victories.

Chie and I squirmed in the back, trying to behave. The talk also connected our down-to-earth concerns with the wider world. They talked about Ikeda-sensei's hope that young people work for peace through Nichiren Buddhism.

We headed home together in the summer dark, insects chirping, fireflies flashing. Elder brother Yusaku proudly led the way; the rest of us bunched behind. As we walked, Dad fixed me in his eyes and said, "Yo-chan, have unlimited dreams. The bigger dreams, the better. Don't be bound by this island's mentality."

The crickets chirped louder. Mom said: "I trust you, Yo-chan."

Like my parents, I am optimistic. If I married a farmer or worked in a factory, I'd still be happy. But an inner voice said, I don't belong here. What awaits out there? I treasured our tiny village; still I left at the first chance.

# PART TWO
# DEPARTURES

A frozen morning
Stable hay is not enough
The grey mare escapes

Colts and phillies
venture forth
spring's exploration

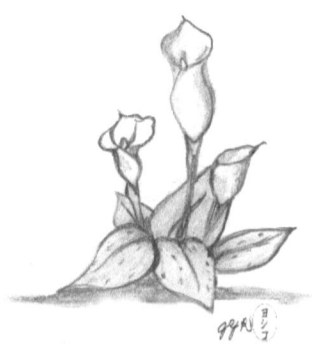

# The Thinnest Hope

## Soka Gakkai Youth Meeting, December 1968

ONCE AGAIN, PETE NEEDED assistance to carry his amps, electric piano, and organ. This time, he didn't need help with a rehearsal. He would perform with a small band for a Buddhist youth gathering at an outdoor amphitheatre near the Santa Monica beach. This time, curiosity overcame scepticism.

The day turned out well for an outdoor event, not hot, under 70 °F. An ocean breeze kept the air fresh and smog-free. Pete and I crammed his equipment into a narrow corner of the stage, amongst the horn section, drum kit, and electric bass. Plenty of time remained before the event began. Pete and the band tuned and adjusted sound levels. I wandered around, checking out the preparations. A chorus and a dance group rehearsed.

Early birds sat on the concrete seats, applauding as others filed in. People came from around Southern California, some alone or in pairs, but many in groups. Nobody my age. A tall guy on stage announced groups in buses from Las Vegas and San Diego to great applause. Wait, I recognize that guy. It's Surfer Larry from Venice. He stepped away from a microphone and leaned towards another guy, passing him a message. Whatever Larry's role, he roved over the stage with the same focus and confidence as I remembered. He looked too busy to say hello, making announcements on the mic and speaking on a walkie talkie. Everyone, the band, dancers, coordinators, even the audience, prepared for a serious production.

As the fifteen hundred-seat amphitheatre filled, they started rehearsing the audience. They handed out balloons and streamers and practised routines.

Noise and enthusiasm filled the event as it began. They sang songs arm-in-arm, waved balloons, cheered for each other.

Everyone, the audience, speakers, and performers, came to be part of an experience. Their message: we are happy and work together peacefully. The entire world can be happy and work together peacefully. Not what I figured to solve world problems, but I didn't lay claim to any better ideas. The gathering came across as close; hokey, but positive.

Balloons and cheers and their rah-rah enthusiasm, at first oddly exciting, wore thin. I needed to clear my head.

I drifted away from the event. On a path outside the amphitheatre, I chatted with a guy who also stepped out from the gathering. Like me, a newcomer. He struck me as a know-it-all, coming across as, "Who do these people think they are? I know about Buddhism." He expected Buddhists to be quieter, more contemplative, and demanded I explain.

I said, "They are a cheerful bunch, but I don't get them either." What the hell am I doing defending this strange group? But this guy's attitude irritated me. Sure, his question was legit, but still. By then, everything and everyone irritated. Can their chanting do something about that?

I made my way back to the amphitheatre and found an empty seat in the back. A short, middle-aged Asian woman on the stage spoke with a heavy accent. Her speech proved hard to follow. She discussed youth and drugs. "You can go on a trip with the drugs, but you always come back to yourself. Back to your apartment and you still must pay rent. Nothing changes. Must change yourself first." Difficult to follow and odd. Why choose a middle-aged woman whose English skills were problematic to lecture a group of young people about drugs?

Her strange presentation made a point, though. Doing drugs made me feel better, but didn't change anything.

A couple of the members told stories of their Buddhist practice. A guy moved from San Francisco, broken by the hippie lifestyle, which was being destroyed by hard drugs and predators. He arrived in LA without hope or direction and found a Soka Gakkai meeting. He joined the same night and, bit by bit, pulled his life together, finding a stable job and reconciling with his estranged family.

Even my damn skin felt sensitive and my arms twitched. But their enthusiasm broke through. I paid attention. They enjoyed the activity and put their excitement on display. Their openness to new ways of living appealed to me. And they showed something I craved — a genuine joy.

Weird, hokey, sure. But sincere. I couldn't criticize. They faced difficulties directly, not complaining about their lives or teachers or parents or society. They didn't wait for a doctor to pronounce they'd spend the rest of their lives in pain or wait for anyone to push a start button.

Their active involvement reminded me of the marches and protests I attended as a kid: the attendants took part, not as a passive audience. They worked together to create the event. Something about their group's commitment felt familiar.

Sick or not, teen angst or not, I resisted giving up on myself. I grasped at the thinnest hope for happiness.

After the meeting, Pete and I tore down his equipment. Pete said, "Let me introduce you to a few people. What did you think of the meeting?"

"I missed part of it. Honestly, it was goofy. Look, if you can teach me how, I'll start today."

Pete, the achiever, the surrogate parent, the ultimate cool jazz musician; once again, Pete's eyes gleamed with tears.

## Learning to chant

At home, we unloaded the equipment. In his room, Pete had arranged a space to chant, with two candlesticks, an incense burner, and a bowl-shaped bell. We sat on the edge of his bed. "Chanting Nam-myoho-renge-kyo taps the wondrous law from the universe outside and from life inside. Everything in the universe is vibrating, you and me, stars, molecules, atoms. Nam-myoho-renge-kyo is like the highest vibration."

"About world peace. You guys spread this for world peace. If that is true, why not convert the most powerful leaders, say Mao Tse Tung, the president, the pope? Three guys and you are done. World peace."

"You've been thinking about this."

"And?"

"Daisaku Ikeda has considered this too. His idea is that lasting change comes from the people, not the leaders. Regular people, not popes and presidents, move history and humanity forward. He wants a thousand individuals to take a single step, rather than three take a thousand steps."

"Who is he? Your god, or something?"

"He's the Soka Gakkai president. Enough talk, little brother . . ."

Pete showed me how to hold the beads from Larry. Then, he lit the two candles and an incense stick and announced we would recite passages from the Lotus Sutra.

He started chanting in a foreign language from a thin blue book. He chanted much too fast for me. The words whirred by in a blur, incomprehensible and unpronounceable. So I hummed along beside him, trying to match his pitch. Soon his room filled with the earthy, evocative sandalwood incense fragrance.

After he finished, he said, "You must learn to do it by yourself, before I leave for Berklee."

"I'll get it. The incense is cool. What's with the beads and candles and stuff?"

"They're accessories. All that's needed is to chant. But they symbolize engaging your senses. We chant with our eyes open, sight. Candles give light. Incense, smell. Holding the beads, touch. The bell, hearing."

"Until you go, can I chant here?" I hoped to use his room once he left.

"Don't touch any of my stuff."

## Giving me room

I started chanting, teaching myself by reading the sutra slowly, while still sceptical of the practice and the group. A few days later, Pete drove me to another meeting at the same North Hollywood house he took me the first time. I still couldn't recite from the book, but followed along, better than before. Pete stood up and introduced me to everyone. Again, his emotion fazed me. I wished to crawl under the rug.

Another man, in his thirties, got up to speak, his stable posture low to the ground, his arms thrown wide, welcoming. He introduced himself as Carlos and spoke in a rich Spanish accent, thick chocolate and cinnamon. He told his experience comfortably, as if speaking to a gathering of dearest friends. As he spoke, he opened his hands and arms smoothly. When he smiled, his entire face smiled.

I imagined Carlos standing in a wood beamed house in front of a sturdy, grained table. Rich tapestries hung on the walls. Dogs munched bones at the foot of a crackling fireplace. Carlos welcomed me and everyone to sit and join him. Let's talk, laugh, sing, and bond.

Despite his engaging demeanour, he told a harsh story, filled with the pain of extreme poverty and discrimination. As the world bore down, he turned to violence.

"My heart filled with hate before I joined. I nearly killed somebody. Convert the hate before it kills you. That's what Nam-myoho-renge-kyo does; I converted rage into music." Carlos, another musician, had a successful studio career.

After the meeting, they hung around chatting. Pete introduced me to Carlos, then left us alone. This is cool; I can talk with this guy alone. Carlos inquired about me, school, Pete mentioned a disease?

"Ninth grade just started. Next year, I hope to get into Fairfax High."

Carlos recommended not to accept anything on blind faith. Practice and study to resolve my doubts myself. Did I play any instruments?

"Not really, not well."

"You've got so much happening. So much inside to come out, so much to contribute. Your family needs you, Keith."

"What's inside is pain. It's called regional enteritis."

"That's your treasure, man, the blessing you bring to the world. That's your song. What made you decide to experiment with the practice?"

"Experiment" sounded reassuring, instead of commit or join or convert or something. He gave me room, and I craved that trust.

Another thing I appreciated — having value now, not potential, not once I got my life together. With Carlos, I didn't pretend to be other than myself, a sick, argumentative, messed up thirteen-year-old. This guy might get me. I told him everything I hadn't even admitted to myself.

"One thing I can see, what I'm doing, isn't working. Faking my way through school no longer works. Most of my friends are gone because of my moves and, honestly, my moods. Dope is taking more and more of my time, and my stomach gets worse. Like you say, I am going to try this. Experiment. I will do it all: the chanting, the meetings, the study, everything. Let's find out what happens. Anything else?"

"Come to our young men's band practice. It's okay if you don't play, just hang out. We gather on Saturdays in Santa Monica. Meet other guys."

The members' energy convinced me to try Buddhism. They demonstrated intelligence, sincerity, commitment, and hope. They didn't meet fewer problems than anyone else, but they appeared to be challenging their problems head on. In some mysterious way, they became happy. Hanging around with older people doing cool stuff felt cool. What did they think of me? Doubtless, I annoyed them.

After Pete left for school in Boston, I moved into his room. To attend the discussion meetings, I rode the bus or hitchhiked. At the gatherings, they shared experiences, introduced newcomers, and studied. Although some of the study bored me, I learned Buddhist principles, philosophy, and history.

Besides the small meetings, the group staged music performances, parades, and festivals. I volunteered for some, learning valuable skills from talented, colourful people. The members came from different backgrounds to work together, pooling their skills amicably. They spoke about challenges at work, home, and in their relationships, and volunteered how their practice helped. They found creative ways to apply the kinds of ideals my family talked about, practising what we preached.

# Siddhartha's Departure

Twenty-five centuries ago, Siddhartha Gautama of the Shakya clan rambled around northern India. He'd left his home, his family, and responsibilities to find a solution to the problem of suffering. What is the purpose of my life, all life? Was I born only to crave, suffer, then die?

After six years of wandering and seeking, he attained enlightenment sitting under a pipal tree. He became enlightened to the dignity of his life, all life, life itself in constant flux, yet bound by causality. He awoke to the life-force of kindness and wisdom.

Siddhartha believed everyone had the same potential for awakening, and he spent the next forty years teaching how. History named him the Buddha, the awakened one. He had troubles and longings and failings and commitment that resonate with me today.

In Siddhartha's time, young noblemen commonly embarked on spiritual quests. They renounced the secular world to go to the forest in search of their enlightenment. That is not what Siddhartha did. From the outset, he looked for a way into life when life itself seemed meaningless.

He sought inner resources — kindness, wisdom, resolve. He looked to engage with his land, its society, the rivers, villages, and highways of northern India. His quest included the political, for we are tied to one another, dependent upon each other, and that is politics. He sought to heal his kingdom, under threat from the outside and broken by a rigid caste system that formalized cruel injustice. And he sought to heal his own broken life, broken by the meaninglessness of suffering and the futility of efforts to relieve suffering.

After his awakening, he painstakingly built a community. He talked, encouraged, laughed, and debated in dusty villages, orderly towns, mango orchards, and bamboo groves. He carried the rain drenched history and fruited destiny of the land, the forests and farms of the Ganges floodplains.

His goal was to live in the world as it is, not as he wished it to be. No prayer, no god would bring his mother back. We will pass, and everything we love will pass. We appear only to disappear. Attempts to impose meaning will pass. The mind constructs meaning, and the mind itself will pass.

I relate to his angst, his discontent, his restless struggle to find purpose amidst suffering. I, too, fear that what I do does not matter, and worse, everything I do may injure others or nature's kingdoms. And I relate to his salvation, not by divine intervention or the birthright of a golden child of destiny, but by a human touch.

Siddhartha Gautama, the sage of the Shakyas, the Buddha, searched for a new way to live. Every human being could turn their greed into giving, their passions into compassion, their delusions into wisdom. I admire his engagement with the creations of humanity to turn them towards serving humanity.

We have something in common, this man who became a Buddha and I. Just beyond our dissimilar stages lies a deeper, shared space, a common landscape of edgy questioning, dissent, and liberation.

Across our stages flesh and blood dramas unfolded; a few I tell here-in. Across millennia and oceans, a web of causality and contingency cradles and links us all. His anguish forced him out: the meaninglessness of an impermanent life driving inexorably to suffering and death. My anguish drove me out. My pain and a vague belief that relief from my pain lay in purpose and purpose lay in my pain.

The word Buddha means enlightened one or awakened one. I use Buddha to refer to the man after he began teaching in Deer Park, near present day Benares, around 445 BCE. I use the name Siddhartha for his time prior. Siddhartha for before he started teaching, Buddha for after.

This is not a historical or authoritative account of his life. These are my speculations based on study and something more: my heart resonates, often awkwardly, occasionally harmoniously, with his childhood, his departure, struggle, collapse, salvation, and eventual awakening. The man called the Buddha, from long ago in India, hails the Buddha in my belly, sometimes whispering, sometimes in a roar: "Fight on."

## Husband and wife, Kingdom of Kosala, 464 BCE

Yasodhara's father's prediction proved true. The arrangements and negotiations between the two families proceeded slowly. Siddhartha's father lacked enthusiasm for a girl from the Koliya clan marrying his only son. He knew Yasodhara's family well and believed them excessively progressive in their views. Yasodhara did not obey the restrictions on young women of their time. He worried that her liberal attitudes would influence Siddhartha.

But Yasodhara's resolve never wavered. Three years after the swan incident, Yasodhara, now sixteen, took Siddhartha as her husband.

For thirteen years they loved each other. They played and belly-laughed and talked. They talked of building a new city, open to every clan and free of superstition. Each person, regardless of caste or gender, would be equal.

For thirteen years they abode in each other, became each other's safe space, each other's forest. They made love in both tempests and infernos. Their chambermaids giggled and whispered: divine lovers plunged to Earth. If no child is born, our Lord and his Lady will cause a new river to flow from the sweat of their exertions. Their families agonized as the couple produced no heir.

And, year by year, Siddhartha's doubts grew. Like a toothache, his primordial angst refused to be ignored. Yes, here he experienced respect, trust, even joy. But, it may not matter. In the end, none of it may relieve the slightest suffering of life on Earth.

Around them society evolved, becoming more uncertain, more dangerous. Empires threatened the Shakyas and other agrarian communities of the Ganges. From the west, the massive Persian empire grew into the Indus valley. From the east, the kingdom of Magadha encroached. Cities replaced country towns. Trade and a merchant class upended agrarian society.

The world evolved in 451 BCE, as it did in 1968, in 2020. As the world does. In changing times, hearts, minds, and behaviour must adapt. Repeating the old ways would no longer work. He shared his discontent with friends, the young elite of the kingdom of Kosala. His friends had studied in Takshashila, the centre of learning a thousand kilometres west. They shared new ideas with Siddhartha, ideas from distant, strange lands: Persia, Greek Bactria, Cīna.

He shared his angst with his Yasodhara, his confident, muse, truest friend. Perhaps he shared too much. Perhaps he scared himself by sharing too much. "If I am to live in this world fully, without suffering," he said to her, "I must do something new, find a new way to think and act."

After thirteen years, he fulfilled his duty to produce an heir for his clan. Now, as a father of a newborn son, Rahula, he considered the future. Every person to come inevitably faced the same fate as every person who came before: birth, misery, death.

## The seamstress, 451 BCE

For years, he considered leaving. Over and over, he shared his doubts and questions with Yasodhara. "The only certainty is death. The time of death is uncertain. What, then, is the purpose of life?"

The morning of their last debate, she visited the clan's garment studio, *paridhaan kaksh*. The seamstress said she'd bring fabric to Yasodhara's quarters, but Yasodhara insisted on taking the newborn to the studio. She'd been confined to home since before the delivery, and craved a few hours of freedom. And, frankly, she sought a fresh perspective on her plight. Rahula nursed or slept while the two women sat amongst fabric bolts, mobile loom, shuttles and wickets, drank tea, and chatted. A shelf by the loom held clay pots filled with dried flowers and saffron for colouring fabric.

The seamstress spoke her mind. "Lady, the city is rife with speculation. They say now that an heir is born, our Lord will abandon the city."

"I fear so. He is determined to pursue his quest. He can be as headstrong as . . . as me. We meet at the second hour after sunset, likely for the last time. *Kakee*, dear, you are my confidente as well as my seamstress. I treasure your counsel as true as your cotton. I will require a new sari to commence my new life."

"Lady Shakya, you are too young to be abandoned alone. Can you not convince our Lord to stay?"

Yasodhara answered, her voice resigned, her eyes darkening grey, a cloud ready to burst. "My husband asks the same questions out loud that we all hold in the hidden, silent corners of our minds. If he stays, he will be miserable, performing daily duties that he believes hurt the people he is to serve. If he leaves and finds nothing, he will bear no regrets. If he leaves and finds answers, we all might benefit."

"In that case, your new-life sari will be yellow to celebrate Rahula's glorious birth, our Lord to be. He carries a bright ray of hope and sunshine for us all. And white, dear Lady, white for peace and purity. You have led a pure, honest life with Lord Siddhartha until now. And you will find peace after he is gone."

Usually so quick with her tongue, Yasodhara took a long time to reply. "Peace, *kakee*? Where is peace in our world?"

"Wear the white, my Lady. You will find peace within. As will he."

## Do not abandon us

At the second hour, they met in the parlour, sitting awkwardly on purple and black cushions, surrounded by lavender curtains. He had not touched her for weeks, other than tenderly holding her hand during Rahula's birth. Their oceanic passion had dissolved into the distant memory of half-forgotten strangers. Whatever he previously desired, he wanted no more. He now desired only not to want. The man she wanted sat nervously across the purple and black settee and a thousand *yojanas* distant.

Yasodhara wore the yellow and white sari prepared by the seamstress, white for her misery, yellow out of respect for their newborn. Rahula slept in the nursery, checked by a maid. Yasodhara refused a wet nurse offered by her father-in-law.

Siddhartha had shaved his beard and hair and wore a holy man's yellow patched robe. The familiar debate tired both.

"If I stay, leading the clan, every day will be a series of duties, rituals, and ceremonies. These tasks are meaningless to me, and worse, lead to more misery for our people. A path out of suffering must lie outside."

Her head wobbled. "Life is not full of suffering. It is full of happiness, with some suffering. The bitter suffering leads to sweeter happiness."

"We say that because of privilege. Others toil in misery for our pleasures. Ignorance mires our clan-folk in the swamps of poverty and disease. As the clan leader, I uphold the very traditions that keep them down. I must find a way for all of us to blossom like lotuses out of the swamp."

"And do you propose to aid the poor and the sick as a forest dwelling monk? What ascetic ever supported the anguished? Ascetics only come out of the forest to harass and beg from poor villagers. You can accomplish much more here, leading your people and teaching Rahula mercy and justice." She lowered her face to hide its frown. *I would have assisted by your side, my Lord. We would achieve so much together.*

"My goal is not to live forever in the forest. Is this world a trap with no escape from discontent? There may be an opening somewhere, a path to freedom, hidden in the forest of prejudice, ignorance, and superstition. If I can find the path, I will return to share it with everyone."

She begged one last time: "Do not abandon us. Do not turn your back on your precious son, your father who loves you, your dear step-mother, who adores you." She begged but did not say please. No tears this time.

"I can not abandon what does not belong to me. You and Rahula are not livestock. He will grow into a fine heir for the Shakyas. My father will ensure your well-being. Everything I own now owns me."

"Everything? Our love? Our dear son? Is he only one more chain restricting your precious freedom?" She'd lost him, recognized it, and no longer cared if her words stung.

"Love? My mother loved me. She died as everybody dies. Father's mighty power couldn't save his own beloved wife. Love is the strongest chain. Love and desire are the jailers, the puppeteer, and the puppet's strings. I must sever the strings from the puppets. For everyone."

"Enough. Halt." She raised her hand as if to slap, but lowered it. She tried to hold his gaze. They both broke; four eyes dropped. She remained silent: You don't speak for "everybody." You claim to wish to end suffering but cause us suffering. You are my Lord and husband, my prince, and my sun and only love. But you disgust me.

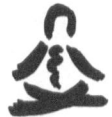

# Students and Teachers

## Student revolts world-wide, 1968–1970

IN LA I ATTENDED schools in white, middle-class neighbourhoods. Mexican-American kids attended my schools. The white and Hispanic kids rarely interacted. We could have been different species occupying the same space.

The schools funnelled students with Spanish surnames into non-mainstream programs. They assigned Mexican-American kids to English as a Second Language programs. Or they placed minority students in vocational programs, or classes for developmentally disabled.

Schools forbade speaking Spanish on campus. These students didn't immigrate to the US. Their families lived in Southern California for three and four generations.

So, the Latino kids in my schools had no access to their own culture and were denied any path to success in mainstream culture. In primarily Mexican-American neighbourhoods, students suffered worse conditions. Under-funded schools on rundown campuses lacked the most basic facilities. Schools did not offer college prep courses. Poorly trained, identifiably racist teachers, taught indifferently.

Mexican-American high school students in Los Angeles protested for better education. Early in 1968, ten thousand students walked out of class. The school boards refused dialogue with their students and called in the police. The police responded with arrests and beatings.[31]

Their protest spread nation-wide and widened across class and racial boundaries.

Between 1968 and 1970, around the world, student protests spread in Tunisia, France, Japan, even behind the Iron Curtain. Young people raged against injustice. Each country's and each school's protest raised their individual issues and causes.

A small group of Japanese schoolteachers founded the Soka Gakkai on Buddhist principles in 1930. Education is in Soka Gakkai's DNA. In the mid-sixties, Ikeda started building non-sectarian schools based on value-creation principles. At the height of the world-wide student protests, in 1969–1970, he'd begun constructing Soka University in Japan.

On January 19, 1969, while hundreds of riot police attacked protesting students at Tokyo University, Ikeda met with a group of students. "Teachers and students should not be in opposing positions. By rights, they are partners walking the path of learning together. Their relationship must be nurturing and democratic. Our purpose is to build a society in which all systems created by human beings contribute to the happiness of humanity and produce genuine value. We must never turn a blind eye to the reality of society."[32]

News of Ikeda's ideas and actions made their way to me. They made sense. The practice and the philosophy and much of the group's actions still made little sense.

Ikeda believed that the same approach could change the self and society: face reality, take positive action, and never give up. "The global rise of student power was, on the one hand, an explosion of the frustration and anger young people felt towards social structures that oppressed and controlled people, and, on the other, a declaration of their rejection of society's established values. The pure spirit of youth exposes the distortions of society like a clear lens."[33]

Now, how do I do that in my life? In some miniscule but real way, my growth could contribute to a more peaceful world. Lasting peace will be created only when people face their warlike tendencies. Changing my situation seemed impossible. Changing society, also impossible.

But working with the guys in band taught me to win in life, to never give up. My life was changing in remarkable ways. The ultimate goal of world peace permeated the Buddhist activities. So the inner shape and the outer began to link, at first in my head, then my body.

That's the movement I yearned to support. Under Ikeda's direction, the activities focussed on making a difference in the world, not about withdrawing from it. When I felt sick and wanted to isolate, not get out of bed, not go to school, one of the guys said, "Keith, this practice works in daily life. If you don't maintain a daily life, it doesn't work."

To me, Ikeda didn't offer panaceas, no cures or solutions, but an approach, a path. The chanting continued to be a mystery, the teachings opaque. But I wanted on that path.

Although still weak and often in pain, I began to find inner strength. The meetings and cultural activities encouraged my growth at home and school and to challenge my weaknesses. No guru or god saved me, but my temperament and behaviour improved. I stopped fighting. I started a school chess club and helped a friend in her campaign for student body office. The simple happiness of being and moving in the world replaced marijuana's euphoria.

In those days, US members of Soka Gakkai travelled to Japan on pilgrimage. When they returned, they taught me more of Ikeda's ideas and his initiatives for peace. I read what I found of Ikeda's writings, translated in the group's US publications. Buddhist history and theory bored or puzzled me, but Ikeda's ideas and his activities spoke to me.

I had more energy, but my stomach didn't improve; the atmosphere at home remained strained. I learned to cooperate from Buddhist activities. But I also had my anger and resentments. Too often, like a bitter old man, I nursed ancient grudges, bent over, clinging to my indignation like a cane, rubbing all the sparkle out of life.

Ikeda spoke to both the world's troubles and mine. I longed to meet him, but the members said I had to be eighteen and healthy for the trip. Anyway, going to Japan cost money and I had none. Too little, too sick, still not enough.

## Band, Santa Monica, 1969

Getting involved in the Buddhist group's activities got me outside of my room and my head. At Carlos' urging, I joined their young men's band. The band performed at events to encourage members and the public, and express their joy of faith through music. Once a week, I travelled by bus to Santa Monica for band practice. As the youngest member and the worst musician, I joined some amazing professional musicians. Others, like me, just wanted to be involved. We came from all sorts of backgrounds and ethnicities. We each had a unique journey with the practice.

Carlos gently, patiently, and generously took me under his care. He led me into mysterious corners of Los Angeles, introducing his anglo protégé to the subtleties of various Latin American cuisines. Super spicy food harmed my stomach. Carlos showed me Latin American foods that were gentle on my stomach.

We sat at a disagreeable looking cantina off of Sepulveda Boulevard devouring cubanos stuffed with pork and fresh cheese. "It's not only tacos and Mexican food, man. There's so much nuance, diversity. These Cuban sandwiches taste mild and deep — no chili peppers, no tortillas. It's like our Buddhism, Keith, so much diversity, for everybody."

Back in Santa Monica, he taught music basics. He explained key signatures using food and cuisine, which I grasped. "Your C major resembles white bread. Basic. Clean." He played the C scales on the piano in the band's practice room. "But if white bread is all you eat, it goes nowhere. It doesn't advance. Then, your minor scales, take G# minor." He played a chord while twisting his lips and face, as if biting into a lime. "See, it has this tang, this suspense, you hear it and you expect something exciting approaching — lime salsa."

Carlos overcame incredible problems in becoming a successful musician and a remarkable teacher. Even today, I have a hard time imagining Carlos being hateful. He cared for me with kindness and strength.

The practice and study directed me inward to a relationship with myself. Chanting became a dialogue, not with an external higher power, but an internal higher me.

To the members of the young men's bands, a note of thanks.

We worked together in common cause despite our differences. I don't know where you guys are today, but I thank every one of you.

Thank you, Carlos, Wayne, Bob, Kurt, Michael, John, and the dozens of others who encouraged me.

You guys accepted me when I didn't accept myself. You taught me to challenge and never quit and how to win at living. I learned to be hopeful by being with hopeful people. I learned to advance instead of complaining by watching you take action for your lives and families and society.

My life today is filled with joy and blessings because of the foundation of faith I learned from each of you. I pray you are well.

# Out There

## Home, 1970

I BORROWED MOM'S POWDER and royal blue Smith Corona Coronet portable and wrote. Too often around others I remained small, inarticulate and intimidated. I skirted the edges, peering in, even in the Buddhist community, never quite feeling I belonged. But I began to view my differences as capabilities, qualities to learn to express. The most improbable idea emerged — those things that made me different, a freak, will be useful to others. Before, I turned to fantasy or defensiveness. Slowly, working with the members of the Buddhist group trained me to be comfortable in the world. Writing met a longing to capture my experience:

```
What it's like, out there: Out there are people who will
harm me, make me feel stupid, make me feel ugly, make me
feel weak.
There are hard people out there, people who know what
they are doing. People who will question what I am
doing. "Why are you here? You don't belong here. What
gives you the right?" People who will say "no."
A part is lost every time I go out there. Some part has
been carved away, stepped on, ripped out, or stolen.
What they want. What they expect. They're gonna take
something from me, take some of me from me.
```

> I know what they say about me, what they think about me, what they already know about me.
> Their face is right in front of me, right up against my face. And I have to say something, and I must do something. And all I can see is them, and their smell is all around me, and their voice is ringing inside me, and I must answer it, and I don't know what to say. And they'll question everything I've done, and make me explain. And they'll judge all that I am. Out there.

## No sense of self, Los Angeles, 1971

> *I no longer had the sense that I was a distinct person.... To be sick in this way is to have the unpleasant feeling that you are impersonating yourself. When you're sick, the act of living is more act than living.*[34]
> Meghan O'Rourke

Impersonating myself. In hindsight, "impersonating myself" fits. I hid behind the masks that got me through the day — the good boy, the rebel, the smarty-pants, the student, the sick kid, the radical, the freak. What else lay behind, other than anger and fear and a sense of being different? Being different is not an identity.

No others with my experience existed. Normal people didn't feel like me. Other people, regular people, didn't pretend to be themselves. Sure, they pretended to be strong or confident or good at climbing fences. But they didn't pretend to be people. Normal people didn't waste time thinking about this stuff.

Of course, I didn't know about a lack of sense of self. I didn't have the words, just the experience. And, since I didn't have any words to understand what I felt, I didn't really experience the experience. I just continued impersonating people I considered normal while rejecting normality.

Without words to describe it, I couldn't feel a loss of self. Instead, I felt anxious and irritated. Since my behaviour was a kind of imitation, I felt whatever I did at any moment was the wrong thing.

Meghan O'Rourke researched and interviewed experts and figured this out in 2013. In 1971, me trying to register for a high school class, Meghan O'Rourke had not been born.

No teacher or doctor or anyone said, hey, you've lost your sense of self, you are impersonating a person. No one resembled me or mirrored my experience. So, I oscillated between attempting to be with others by pretending better and rejecting others by rebelling better.

My loneliness became more than not having friends or even being alone. My loneliness became a deep comprehension that nowhere in the universe existed a person with whom I'd connect.

O'Rourke wrote of those with compromised immune systems: "In your loneliness, your preoccupation with an enduring new reality, you want to be understood in a way that you can't be."[35]

Being denied that I was sick made me feel like I was not myself. The fall from denied, nameless illness to unseen illness to concealed identity to denied self was not, of course, exclusive to me, nor to kids with Crohn's. Ninety-four percent of disabled Americans lack visible signs such as wheelchairs or canes.[36] In an article in the AMA Journal of Ethics, Dr. Jennifer Dobson discusses invisible illness:

> *Lack of empathy from clinicians can leave patients feeling misunderstood, isolated, and that they must bear the burdens of their disease without help. Some clinicians express frustration with patients with illnesses of presently invisible etiology—blaming them, resenting symptoms without the privilege of certain expression, accusing them of being dishonest or 'difficult,' pathologizing them as malingering or psychosomatic, or labeling them in ways that are dismissive of their deep knowledge and understanding of their own bodies and lived experiences. Such dismissals are common...*[37]

The shadow people aren't insane, but they might think they are and might be treated as such.

## Sense of purpose

Throughout childhood, I had a sense of not being real. I took an uncertain first step into the classroom of grade one, three days after school had started and fifteen minutes late. The other kids were already seated. They knew how to sit, how to be students, the actual students. I spotted a kid from my street, 34 Avenue, in Kerrisdale. He sat at a desk. Behind him sat an empty chair. I headed for it, but the teacher stopped me. "Oh, we prepared a seat for you. You sit there." She pointed to the other side of the room. I blew it, first day of school. The other kids could see: I can't even sit right. I got the message: this is how school will be.

As I grew older, people told me, "Oh, you are young; you are blessed with so much potential." They intended to encourage and praise. That's not how I took it. I heard "not good enough. Not worthy, yet." One day, if I became different, and realised my potential, I'd be enough. Later, once my life started.

Waiting in a spinach-green curtained cot to be released from quarantine or for a doctor to define what my body is doing. Waiting for the wizard to arrive and push my start button. Start my life. Once it starts, my stomach won't hurt. That's what ailed my stomach; my life hadn't started. I'd yet to begin the serious business of being a person.

In a restaurant, I'd glance at the other tables. Those people sitting, feasting, they are real diners, the type of people who dine at restaurants, this kind of restaurant. I rode a bus most every day. I'd examine the other riders and think, those are the bus riders. That's what bus riders do; the real bus riders read the paper, or chat, or stare out the window.

After I started chanting and studying Buddhism, things started moving. My stomach didn't improve, but at least my illness had been acknowledged. It proved real. And, dammit, I stumbled forward. With the pain and the fatigue, sure I couldn't do everything, but I did some things. My attendance at school improved. I made new friends. And I ceased taking drugs as I grew both calmer and more energetic, more in the world and less eager to escape.

I attributed my growth to my Buddhist practice and activities. But chanting wasn't an abracadabra magic formula. My practice existed in a context, a framework of a movement for peace based on personal transformation. The shape of that, the directionality, came from Ikeda. The organization published translations of his speeches and lectures. His poem "Ode to Youth," like Carlos' encouragement, planted a seed that my misery could become a sense of purpose:

> *I have a mission uniquely my own.*
> *You too have a mission like that of no other,*
> *For without the vigorous energy of youth,*
> *what can be done for our feeble age?*
> *The slope of construction,*
> *from rough-hewn to perfection,*
> *The song of youth,*
> *The rhythm of culture.*
> *Now, sounding the gong of reformation*
> *Let's work on bravely through the rain.*[38]

Ikeda lived five thousand miles away, speaking and writing in a foreign language, putting his trust in the world's youth. Soka Gakkai had millions of members world-wide. Technically, I remained outside the millions, not old enough to join formally. Across these divides we connected, as though a gong he sounded vibrated a cord buried in me. I wanted to reciprocate and reply to his trust. I had no interest in becoming his fan or idolising him.

Another factor attracted me to Ikeda. As I write in 2022, he is in his nineties. He's struggled with ill-health most of his life. As a youth, he had tuberculosis. Through wartime and postwar Japan he was too poor to afford a sanitorium. The doctors proclaimed he would not survive past thirty. He wrote, "The experience of illness makes us more compassionate. Illness teaches us many things. It makes us look death in the face and think about the meaning of life. It makes us realize just how precious life is."[39]

He identified with those who were suffering. He stood on my side. So, I longed to be on his.

Slowly, I learned responsibility around the house and for my health, school, happiness. I needed to be responsible to my mentor as well, not to enter a childlike, passive dependency. I yearned to connect with him, person to person.

Maybe I could be real. Maybe, even with Crohn's, I'd plan for university, find a girlfriend, and create a future. Like normal kids. Simple. I had to meet him.

## US literature, history, culture

The room shook. The bed bounced. Mom yelled, "Get under the doorframe. Earthquake!" The shaking continued for almost a minute.

The 1971 Chatsworth earthquake spared our house and Fairfax High from severe damage. But Fairfax became impacted. The earthquake destroyed Fairfax's neighbour, Los Angeles High School. So, students at LA High took classes in the afternoons at Fairfax. Fairfax High classes shifted to mornings.

I attended Fairfax because I studied Russian. The earthquake put my continuing school at Fairfax in doubt.

Letters came in the mail from the Board of Education and from Fairfax High regarding lack of space because of the earthquake. They announced I might not continue at Fairfax, that studying Russian alone might not be enough. They might transfer me in the middle of the last semester of grade 11 to the closer school.

Mom pulled out the Coronet to write scathing letters back and to the State Superintendent of Schools and the Governor and whomever. "Mom, wait, I've got a couple of ideas."

First idea: chant. Second: Two teachers at Fairfax started a pilot class combining American history with culture. Traditional history, art, and literature classes taught the elements of society in isolation. In the new class, students would learn the ways history and culture influenced one another. That remained where my interest lay: study history to find connections.

More than American history, I wanted to learn my context, if I fit into the world.

I enjoyed studying history. The names of kings or dates of battles were boring. Discovering the ways things connected wasn't boring. The pain of my isolation created my longing for connections. If my future had any hope of differing from my past, I needed to find out how we arrived at the present. I'd learned little of my history, family, or culture. Outside school, I read books on history, the Holocaust, African history. Books on escapes fascinated me — the Underground Railroad, escapes from prisons, concentration camps. History meant forming connections and shattering chains.

Since the class was experimental and new, no other school offered anything similar. If I got into the class, they might let me stay at Fairfax. A student in the program, the sensitive, brilliant, delectable Evelyn Payne, told me the class required more students. She said the new compressed schedule and now overcrowded classes threatened the new program. They needed students. I needed to stay in Fairfax. The possibility of being in class with Evie became a bonus. All right, an equal draw.

## Teacher's lounge, Fairfax High School

Outside the building, heavy equipment banged and rumbled. Workers set up Quonset huts and trailers for the students coming from LA High. Dust and smog clouded the air.

The teachers' lounge was usually off-limits to kids, a place I didn't belong.

The scent of stale coffee and popcorn greeted my entrance. Several stacks of new books sat on a corner of a stained banquet table, wobbly with mismatched legs. Two men faced me, next to the stacks, with papers and file folders spread in front. Young-ish for teachers, the one with a military crew cut hairstyle wore a sweater vest. The other wore glasses and a brown elbow-patched tweed jacket. Both of their ties hung askew, loose at their collars.

Today's interview was compulsory for acceptance into the course. I scanned the room. A battered percolator sat on a counter. Notes and signs hung from a corkboard. Tired furniture dotted the room. I searched for hints to whom they sought to admit. Through the dirty windows, workers set up trailers for temporary classrooms.

The crew cut teacher introduced the experimental course. He portrayed it as innovative. Nothing else compares. Their professional reputations put at stake. He sipped out of a chipped mug. He leaned on the table, and its wobble startled the other teacher. Post earthquake jitters.

Tweed jacket removed his glasses and wiped them with his tie. "Keith, tell us about your interest in American history and culture."

"Well, um, history is the manner we got here. If we want to understand who we are, we must study what led here. What are the causes of the country's problems? I want to develop who I am and contribute to social justice. To create a different future, uncover what created the present. Connections, how things fit." I sure hoped I'd fit in with the class.

Crew cut sipped more coffee. "We accept students who are up to the challenge of the course and material." Outside, a jackhammer pounded. Tweed jacket jumped again.

"Sorry?"

"As long as we are talking history, your records show difficulty getting along at your previous schools. This course is not for slackers. The workload will be heavy. We expect the highest commitment from our students. Whether the course succeeds depends on those who attend. We will hold the students to our high standards."

The moment arrived, demanding courage I lacked. I stammered: "I've been doing things differently. Won't have those problems here. I put down dope. Now practising Buddhism, chanting." Stronger: "Tell more about your new class. You said innovative?"

Get them off me. Encourage them. And it worked; away they went, elaborating on concepts, curricula, talking over each other, excited. My stomach still hurt, but that wasn't new.

Their excitement triggered my excitement. Now, get in there, give this everything: "I've been making changes so that I can contribute. I want in this program to uncover the connections between culture and history. But also, so I can connect, so I can be part of the American experience. My spiritual mentor taught that human beings and culture drive history, that youth must create a new age of peace. I require this class to become like that. Learning from your program is important."

They accepted me into the course. I bought copies of Richard Hofstadter's *The American Political Tradition*, Arthur Miller's *The Crucible*, and a literature anthology.

On the bus home, I began reading Hofstadter: "...the traditional ground is shifting under our feet. It is imperative at this time of cultural crisis to gain fresh perspectives on the past."[40]

## Chanting

When I arrived home from the interview, I headed straight for Pete's room, my room while he studied in Boston. I kept the chanting space in the corner. A bell and mallet sat on the floor next to a cushion. A coffee table held two candles and a rectangular incense burner half-filled with ash. I cleared space on the table for the three books for the class, stacking them neatly, Hofstadter on top. I lit the candles and incense, then opened the doors to the little nut-brown altar he'd hung on the wall, sat on the cushion, and, holding the beads Larry gave me, began evening prayers.

Nam-myoho-renge-kyo. Nam-myoho-renge-kyo. Accepted into the history program. Thanks. Thanks to who or what doesn't matter; it's gratitude.

Nam-myoho-renge-kyo. Next, to study and learn the ways culture and history wind together. How they connect. The role a single person can play. The role I might play. First, learn the connections. Here I am.

Nam-myoho-renge-kyo. Here I am, chanting, praying, thanking. Whoever I am, wherever I came from, is here now. This is me. Now. Entire me. Every one of "me" is here — student, son, utility outfielder, crappy chess player, brother.

Settling into the chanting, I rub the beads between my palms. For the moment, my stomach is quiet. I pick up the pace. Nam-myoho-renge-kyo.

My history, known or not, is here, present. Everything I've said and done is here, now. Everything. Fights after school. Bloody faces. Can't remember the names. A quiver of shame, I raise my hands to my face, heat comes off my cheeks. An old hospital room reeking of Betadine and floor disinfectant. The savoury flavours of Mom's Hungarian stuffed green peppers. The smell of the grass and my glove's leather, and the sound of the ball landing in the mitt, and that clear, beautiful "Out!" from the umpire. Sensei's writings on revolution without violence. Seeking something new, my revolution, not out there, in here. In this me.

A flutter in my belly. I take a breath. The sensation ripples up into my chest. Continuing the chanting, now with determination. Don't miss band practice. Twenty minutes a day, study the sutra. Study Hofstadter and connect the threads of my life, my history. Support Mom and Dad so they don't argue so much. Be fully part of this family. Create something new. Nam-myoho-renge-kyo. Nam-myoho-renge-kyo. This is me. With this body. With this family. Here. For the briefest moment, a sense — welcomed in this place, attentive, upright and alert. As if a golden capsule enclosed and emanated from me. A brief sensation that immediately floated away. Here I am. Bowing, I rang the bell to finish.

# Siddhartha's Quest

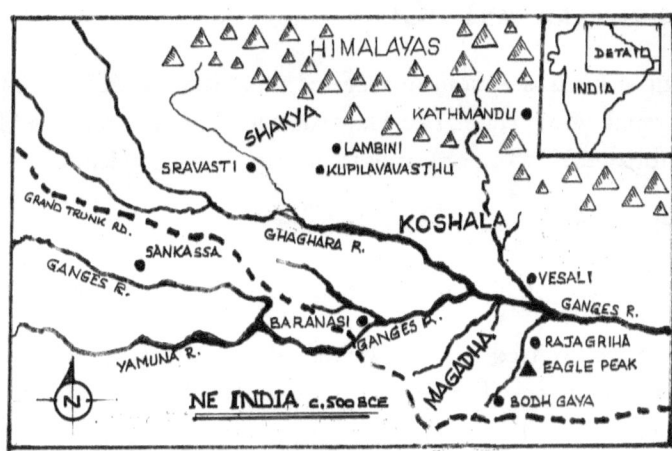

Map courtesy of Black Pearl Film Works

SIDDHARTHA'S INDIA WAS EVOLVING. Expanding trade led to power shifting to the commercial classes. Practical and cosmopolitan, traders rejected the rigidity of Brahmanism. New philosophies and new social structures emerged.

He sought a new way to live, and a new way to live together. At home he'd be leading his small clan through major crises and petty squabbles. His life, inevitably, would be conservative, protecting old ways. Clan responsibilities and rituals left little room for philosophical explorations. He had to go out.

He set off, ill prepared for the dangers of the road. Wearing the robe he'd fashioned, he carried the copper razer he'd used to shave his head and a bowl for begging. The monsoons finished. The last debate with Yasodhara finished. He marched to the Great Northern Road that crossed his town of Kapilavastu.

Then he turned east on the still muddy highway. The roads were dangerous, particularly through forests. Forests held bandits, tigers, bears. For safety, he negotiated passage on caravans. Walking with the caravans could lead to meeting other seekers, learning about distant lands, and discovering new ideas. Another seeker may be on the same search, a step or more ahead of him. His quest would not remain solitary.

## The caravan, 451 BCE

The first captain, sceptical, interrogated him: "Safe passage comes at a price, Shakyan. Nobody travels free. Have you coin? Chippies for trade? Do you read fortunes? Do you cast spells to protect against accidents?"

"I seek a path to liberation for everybody."

"And you, are you liberated or enslaved, enlightened or common?"

"There are no fixed selves, enlightened or benighted. Only in action does virtue or wickedness surface or drown. Only in adversity does one's strength arise."

"Hmm. Your speech differs from the usual claims of holiness and purity from yellow-robed drifters. But you're young. You haven't found your path, let alone mastered it."

"Sir Captain, do not err by dismissing the young: a fire while still a spark can expand to burn your stores and carts and feed. The venom of a baby snake kills as surely as its grandfather's. A young prince on the throne can raise armies to blockade your highways. And if you impede a virtuous seeker on his quest, you risk remaining childless, your manhood soft as the rotting stump of a dead palm tree."

"Hah." The captain chortled. "You win, Lord Shakya. Join my caravan and entertain with your curses and riddles. I can use a noble-born, trained in mathematics and law. Many try to trick me, twist my books and skim the receipts. You will mind the scales of the feed merchants. While you search for your path, earn your keep by sifting the straight from the crooked."

Around the night fire, the two talked. The captain drank *masara* from the west, when available, or *bhang*, cannabis in a thin yogurt drink. He provided rich information on the changing world. He'd seen it all — floods and elephant stampedes and troops of archers marching west to sell their deadly services to the Persian Emperor. With gusto, he shared his tales of the women and the drink of distant lands.

"Captain, you consider yourself a devotee of Shiva, the Auspicious One?"

"Aye, Shakyan, of course. The vedas teach moderation in drinking. Since I follow Lord Shiva, I can moderately drink *masara* and moderately drink *bhang*, then the same of *thandai*. Treble the moderation."

"My concern is the misery of this world, not your drink. It seems only an evil god creates a world full of evil, of suffering. A god capable of creating this world must have left an escape, a path to freedom."

"You may find it, yet. On my highway or off. That day you become *devâtideva*, the Teacher of Gods."

On the highway, Siddhartha listened to the hopes and troubles of those he met. Each person on the road had a history, a regret, and unattainable cravings. Each told their story, be they domestic slave, proud noble, or washer-woman cleaning the robes of the travelling lords and ladies. He spoke with traders fretting over delivery delays and anxious farmers hauling crops to cash markets. World-weary teamsters drove the carts ever eastward towards the mouth of the Ganga. Ever-weary prostitutes traipsed behind the train. They sold their bodies to others' desires, while longing for their mothers and homes.

Like a city in motion, with hundreds of carts, the caravan ground across northern India, running roughly parallel to the sacred Ganga. Spanning miles, the train conveyed sugar, jewellery, oils, embroideries, furniture, perfumes. The stuff of life transported from trade port to port, train halt to train halt. They carried new products — spices from the south, textiles and pearls from Persia, even rolls of silk and pieces of jade from as far as Cīna. Different ways of living. And new ideas.

Not just cargo and travellers, the caravan carried livestock and hundreds of work animals. Horses from central Asia were the main livestock of trade. Elephants, of course, and the occasional rhino. Once, the train carried a tiger for a prince in southern Pandya. But only once. Three nested cages mounted on wheels held the wild beast, who spent every waking moment of the journey struggling to be free. The day and night roars, growls, and snarls reverberated up to a *yojana* away, keeping the entire train sleepless and in fear. The captain lost more income from terrified merchants withdrawing their freight.

No tigers and no slaves. Household slaves travelled on the caravan with their owner-families, of course. But the captain refused to haul slaves for trade. He heard that in the far west, the toga robed barbarians bought and sold humans in slave markets. Not on his train. Anyway, plenty of people sold themselves freely; not necessary to import savages from uncivilised western lands.

Farmers and merchants with market vegetables and livestock joined the train to supply the demands of the caravan itself. The captain and his bookkeepers kept careful track of prices and transactions. They received strange coins from distant lands used for trade. Siddhartha kept careful track of the bookkeepers and the scales.

The caravan attracted the usual grifters, faith-healers, and fortune-tellers. These charlatans haunted the roads and preyed like hawks on innocent travellers. The captain ran a clean train and refused to accept a slice of their dirty pickings. He saw no contradiction with his own beliefs in prophecy and curses. Siddhartha protected the train and travellers by hunting the hustlers, exposing their flim-flams.

Besides the con artists, the only others Siddhartha wouldn't tolerate were the priests. Well, they were just another type of grifter. He debated any Brahmin priest who had the courage to face his wrath in public. "Instead of sacrificing innocent beasts to your gods," he'd argue, "sacrifice yourself for the sake of the poor. Instead of your rituals of obedience, live with kindness."

## The music of the universe

Minstrels tagged along the train. The caravan halted for weather or accidents, poor roads, or auspicious days on the calendar. Out the minstrels would jump, playing zithers, fifes, and *maram* drums. Travellers gathered to dance and sing along to their songs of losses in love and victories in war and harvests and old gods.

Siddhartha recalled the dancers and musicians his father hired to entertain at court. In the evenings Siddhartha and Yasodhara had enjoyed strolls in the gardens around the clan house. They'd return home to find entertainers performing for the nobles. Night after night the wealthy nobles drank and were entertained by musicians, singers, and dancing maidens. Often servants carried the nobles to their beds.

Siddhartha quickly bored of the routine. One evening, just before the Shivarati festival, the partying grew intense. On the festival night itself, worshipers fasted and prayed and refrained from intoxicants. So they indulged prior. The nobles consumed pitcher after pitcher of *maireya*. The entertainers also became intoxicated on *bhang*, Lord Shiva's divine cannabis. Young female chorus members danced with the noblemen.

All royal youth received classical training in music. He asked Yasodhara, "Darling, are you enjoying the festivities?"

"Not very much," she answered. Like her husband, she tired of such entertainment. And she knew his ambivalence towards the gods.

"I like music," said Siddhartha, "it is beautiful. It is natural to be attracted to something beautiful. A harmless satisfaction. But over and over brings on a kind of sickness. Satisfaction turns to boredom. A boredom sickness."

"Let's stroll in the gardens, dear. Leave the faithful to their festivities."

They enjoyed each other's company far more than his father's entertainments. "The performers are human beings first. Yasodhara, do you think they are happy singing and dancing and making music for us?"

"This is their livelihood and support for their families. Your father treats them well. They are not abused as elsewhere."

"So, it is all performance, a masquerade? And we are to pretend we enjoy it?"

"They are talented and trained. I am certain they enjoy both creating music and satisfying their audience. When they tire, they drink intoxicating beverages."

"And Lord Shiva, the Beneficent, instead of helping the miserable, wants us to drink and party in His honor? And then, on His night, the Shivarati, we are to fast and pray and be pious?"

"Dear husband, the evening air chills. Let's return to our home."

The couple arrived home to a shock. The celebrations had ended. Both the entertainers and nobles, even the servants lay about, intertwined sleeping on pillows. They had all passed out from drink and revelry. The couple stepped around the prostrate bodies. In sleep, their beautiful joyous faces looked ashen and drawn. Their fancy make-up now smeared like garish paint; their elaborate costumes now wrinkled, stained, and worn. The young ladies of the chorus looked even younger, mere children lying amongst adults.

In sleep, all their differences disappeared. Caste, gender, and roles became meaningless to the unconscious. The hour was late, long after dusk. He and Yasodhara were tired. He had a strange thought, like a foreign voice in his mind. Was it a whisper from the god Shiva? "You, too, are asleep. This is all your dream. You must awaken. Hurry."

Back in the caravan, the music of the highway rang fresh to his ears. The minstrels' songs captured both the present moment and the passage of time through months and seasons and generations.

They played sacred music, earthly music, the tragic and ribald. He heard the elements of the universe — water dripping and crashing, wind howling, fire roaring, the earth's hum, thunder booming. Whether a lighthearted children's song or a pained ode to lost love, the music pulsed through his ears, vibrating his bones and blood. The chords, complex or simple, climbed scales like rungs of a ladder into an arpeggio of joy, an ode to the energy and richness of being.

Many of the musicians and entertainers on the highway were of the third gender, called *kinnars*. Excluded from the rigid structures of caste and gender, some had been ruthlessly exploited. Some *kinnars* had been branded or mutilated, forced into harems as eunuchs, or toys of the privileged. Now they followed the highways, eking out the barest living as travelling minstrels. Through music, they expressed their inner ecstasy. Sitting with them, learning their stories, reminded Siddhartha of his unease at the musicians performing at court. Now, hearing the *kinnars'* joy in the face of lifetimes of abuse, Siddhartha's eyes opened to new possibilities. Many ways to live were possible. Despite overwhelming impediments, they lived with laughter and generosity. Despite the cruelty of others, they lived with joy.

He silently vowed to remember them; the path must include everybody. Each one liberates themselves by thoughts and actions, their music, not from gender or position.

And the *kinnar* minstrels didn't forget him. Over forty years later, at Eagle Peak near Magadha's capital, he taught the Lotus Sutra for everyone. The *kinnars* gathered at the assembly to testify for him. Appearing as heavenly singers and dancers, the *Kimnaras*, they pledged to protect the wonderful dharma and its teacher.

Witnessing fellow travellers' blooming joy in dance and song filled him with hope, renewed his determination. Whatever it required, no matter the impediments, he must find his answers. If no way existed, he'd clear a path and construct the road himself.

## The countryside

He sought gurus in the countryside who offered answers. So, he left the caravan outside Rajagriha. Bidding the captain farewell, he said, "If I find a dharma to end anguish, Captain, your trains will carry it to the world."

"Lord Shakya, I am just a lecherous old drunk. You will be the first *Maha-sarthavaha*, the Great Caravan Leader of the World. Your steps will create the highway of our deliverance."

Off the highway, he slept in ditches with tramps. Or he negotiated nights in barns with farmers, protecting their chickens and goats from pythons and monkeys. In villages and towns, he studied the crafts of carpenters and smiths. "Why does a holy man study road and house building?" queried a construction crew chief.

"What I don't find, I must raise myself. I must learn the principles of construction." Siddhartha'd never forgotten his childhood vision of discovering an ancient city in the forest.

So, carpenters showed how to work a plumb and line. Before masons laid the first un-moulded sun-baked bricks, the foundations and outline must be straight and sure. Whatever he built demanded to be sturdy and flow in straight lines toward the future. In a smith's noisy workshop, he learned the value of balancing heat, the power required to shape metal.

For all his anxiety over whether any of our actions matter in a world whose only certainty is the end, survival mattered to those he met. Their families mattered; having food to ride out the rainy season mattered. Love and children and sex and dramas and traumas and clan feuds and the price of Ceylonese tea, and whether monkeys stole their hen's eggs, or a python devoured their goats, mattered. And they found simple joys in their toil and in one another. He intended his quest for everybody. If he genuinely considered people as living, struggling, tormented beings, what mattered to them, best matter to him.

## The realm of pure spirit

Siddhartha studied, practised, and debated with the top gurus of both the old Vedas and newly emerging philosophies. On the highways, travellers told of a great yogic holy man, Alara Kalama. They said he had attained a state of nothingness and oneness with the god Brahma. Siddhartha travelled to Alara's hermitage outside the city of Vaishali. Alara meditated undisturbed by the rumble of carts on the road outside his hermitage. He took this as proof of his great spiritual achievement.

Siddhartha became Alara's disciple and soon mastered the meditation. He entered a state where matter dissolved into raw spiritual emptiness. Alara suggested Siddhartha join him in leading his group. But mastering nothingness did not resolve his persistent unease. He blocked out earthly concerns, but the carts still rolled outside, the wheel of suffering kept turning.

Alara meditated as a goal. But Siddhartha meditated as a technique, a means to freedom. Alara's meditation became an end to enter a state beyond the limits of the fleeting mind and beyond the mud and muck of life. Even if the goal was desirable, only a precious few could achieve it.

Alara's technique didn't offer a solution to anguish. Siddhartha sought a way for every person to express their highest capacities, not to escape their joys and struggles. He looked for a practice by which regular people liberated themselves from the chains of anger, ignorance, and cravings. The liberation he sought must be within daily life, with all its instability and loss.

In the end, Siddhartha thought, "Their teachings left me unsatisfied. I left Alara and went away." The mindless pursuit of ever more treasure led only to increased discontent. Escape in spiritualism and promises of after-lives did nothing for the sufferings of today. A path into life and out of misery must lie somewhere. There must be a path to inner freedom, a path available to every sentient being.

In a 1988 speech, Daisaku Ikeda discussed inner freedom: "Freedom is not found somewhere apart from the seeming constraints . . . of life's realities. Nor is true freedom found in escaping reality. Where is there to escape to? We can't escape from the universe. And more important, we can't escape from our own lives." [41]

The Ganges flood plain's fertility allowed people to live beyond just survival. New ways of living required new ways of thinking.

## Failure and failure

He rejoined the road, trailing the wheels of the wagons traversing northern India. Bullock carts carried produce raised by the hands of farmers, wooden goods made by artisans, fabrics hand spun on spindle whorls. The beauty of the ordinary produced by living hands. The self is not independent of its environment; the spirit cannot separate from the flesh. Holiness is in the labour of hands, prayer in every knot tied in the fisher's net. The potter meditated every turn of the wheel, their hands on the clay in prayer. Siddhartha sought answers in human creations, not in the gods'.

For six years he trekked the Gangetic plain, on and around the Great Northern Road. Legends say that for six years he practised extreme asceticism, that each day he consumed a single grain of rice, one sesame seed, and one drop of water. This seems improbable as historical fact. The legends fit too neatly into the model of a superhuman spiritual recluse. More likely for six years, he studied, discussed, debated, meditated, and thought.

But nothing changed. His wandering had not brought him a single step closer to resolving his anguish. All his efforts and debates helped no others. His vow to lead people to freedom became an empty promise. Talk and ideas alone did not provide meaning. Life remained destined to suffering, causing suffering to others and death.

He roamed the pumpkin orange, russet, and green patchwork of fields, forests, and rivers. He possessed a patched yellow-ochre robe, a knife for shaving, and a beggar's bowl. Along the way, he'd lose the bowl and knife. Time and abuse reduced the robe to rags. Certainly, he lived on the edge. Step by step and year over year, he grew thinner, weaker. As certainly, he did not spend six years in an ascetic near-death meditative trance.

Over the years, his thinking evolved, became clearer. His years of study before the departure and six years of discussions and debates informed his language and methods later when he taught. But, at the time, his ideas helped not a single anguished soul. His own angst persisted without relief. Nothing eased his pained concern for the pain he witnessed everywhere.

Desperate now to resolve his angst, he joined five ascetics who practised extreme self-denial. They believed the only way to end the sufferings of the self must be to end the self, free the spirit by denying the body. His own body weakened further.

Self-denial caused him to crave simple comfort and connection. The more he repudiated the self, the more self-conscious he became. Denying his body made it more demanding of sustenance. Denying sensation created more longing for feeling.

For six years, he searched and failed. Every path led to a dead end. Every practice and discipline and philosophy led nowhere. What a waste. His efforts remained in vain. More vanity. Just another wandering, hungry beggar.

# My Quest

### Santa Monica, Early 1971

I HEARD IKEDA PLANNED to visit America in 1972. This news thrilled me. Finally, the chance to meet my teacher.

The group began preparing for his visit. After one Saturday practice, Carlos spoke to a few guys in the band. His shirt, as always, tucked straight, his curly hair trimmed short. "He won't be preaching. Sensei is coming to encourage us in everything — work, family, health, life. We've got a lot to prepare, gonna be together with him, baby, breathing the same air, chanting and dancing and playing on the same stage. We'll be making music together, man, creating our masterpiece."

Groups in each city on his itinerary scheduled local festivals. The celebrations would culminate in a general convention in Los Angeles in May, 1972, with thousands attending. The members needed to organize, write, and rehearse music and dance performances. Stages and sets needed construction; thousands of costumes sewn. And chanting, lots of chanting, individually and in groups, large and small. We would celebrate the joy of our experience with the practice and show how people might work together in peace. The largest event was planned for Los Angeles.

This was it. The biggie. The sole chance to meet my mentor, show him my report card, the improving grades, tell him my anger turned to positive energy. Ideally, I'd report that my family fought less; perhaps Mom and Dad could meet him. I had no wider knowledge of his plans or schedule; as far as I knew, there'd be no second chance.

Juggling studies and schedules, I'd dive in all the way. I wished to join the stage crew, hammer nails, run cables. They seemed a groovy crew; get in with them, if I could. If not, it didn't matter. Support whatever way. Work with cool people. Fun. Pull all-nighters.

Soon after preparations began cranking up, Dad had news. He would take a sabbatical to Israel and Europe. With me. For a year, including during Ikeda's visit to LA. This news did not thrill me. It crushed me.

I'd attended peace rallies with tens of thousands of protesters. I'd been to love-ins in Griffith Park, listened to (and fell in love with) Janis Joplin. But this event with Ikeda differed from the others. It was going to be . . . important. And I had to leave to be with my bickering parents. A year without school, travelling the world. Sounds good, right? Not to me. Too old for a tantrum, I argued, bargained.

Life has disappointments. I experienced plenty. But missing these activities implied more, a waste of my chance at wholeness. Missing this opportunity meant I didn't deserve opportunities.

In my mind, meeting Ikeda became a longing deeper than any hunger. I lacked the words — fulfilment, redemption for all my failures, for the projects I started and never finished. My obsessive nail biting and skin picking, tearing my skin until bloody and infected. Quitting the piano. Leaving the sprinklers on and flooding Mom's garden. Her saying I became "the best rationale for birth control." Overeating. Being empty and naked and held up by the scruff of my neck for everybody to examine and ridicule. Having broken guts.

But, like water trapped underground, a dimly felt sense of worth seeped into my consciousness. Even my unhappiness remained part of my worth. The singularity of my misery might encourage another.

Fine, this is me. This package of pain and teen angst and oddness is who I am. Nobody else suffered in precisely my way. So, my purpose existed in my anguish, something I must do, that only I can do.

Naïve and idealistic, I was, oh yes. Still am. But no hero-worshipper. Ikeda couldn't fix these things, couldn't fix me. I knew that. But I became convinced that to fulfil my purpose, I had to meet him.

## Meeting with Larry

The new school year approached. We needed to plan my accommodations. Still a minor, I could not stay at home alone. And I had to finish high school at some place. Dad's sabbatical started in September, when my final year of high school was starting. Unlikely I could finish high school in Israel. One way or the other, I would be leaving home. I would be going out there, whether I tagged along with Mom and Dad or stayed behind somewhere.

---

I met with Surfer Larry to inform him of my dilemma. He worked at Soka Gakkai's Santa Monica center. I sought backing for my plan, not advice. We met in a simple room, fluorescent lights, folding chairs across from each other. On two walls hung frames with mysterious oriental calligraphy. Boxes stacked on the floor against another wall, with newspapers and office supplies.

"I'm being punished. All I want is to meet sensei." My plan: "I can stay with friends and finish high school. My uncle can arrange groceries. I need an adult to act as a guardian."

"How old are you?"

"Seventeen this year."

Fortunately, Larry was an adult. "Keith, you can't live on your own in LA. LA is too much for a sixteen-year-old alone. Actually," Larry paused, lips slightly parted, eyes intense now, two drills boring into me, "LA can be too much for anyone. You must go with your family."

Crushed again. "You don't understand my parents."

For a moment, the cool surfer's eyes clouded. "I get it. I get it. You don't know mine." He continued, his eyes clear again, his voice determined, "Your parents are alive. What about taking care of them? Remember, you and I are practising to expand our lives and create happy families. It is hard work." And then, "Think about it, Keith: thousands of members from all over will be here. Realistically, the chances of you personally meeting sensei are slim."

Realistically. There's that word. The tiniest pin prick exploded the thin balloon of my hopes.

Larry continued. "You won't miss him. Next April, go to Paris."

Larry wrote an address on a scrap of paper, an address in Sceaux, France. "I can't read this."

"It's in Paris, Keith. Or near. You'll need to look it up. April, next year."

## Spain, Early 1972

In the end, they left without me. Dad had to be at a university in Haifa, Israel, in September. I had to finish high school in Los Angeles. So, I took summer school in 1971 and moved in with friends in September. My uncle, a Navy lawyer, picked up cases of canned goods for my meals at a US military trading exchange. With an extra load of classes in September, I accumulated just enough credits to graduate in January 1972. The plan I'd presented to Larry sort of materialized.

In January 1972, I flew to join my parents in Israel. For months, we travelled around Israel, North Africa, and southern Europe. Our yellow Volvo station wagon proved too large for the narrow roads of Moroccan medinas and the villages of Franco's fascist Spain. Mom and Dad often quarrelled. I sat in the back, on the trip of a lifetime, in a teenage sulk. Dad focussed on his current assignment, or whatever project came next. Mom fulfilled her dream of travelling to the homes and beds and battlegrounds of the Greek gods and goddesses. I obsessed over finding sensei on my own, surviving, not screwing this up.

In Andalucia, Spain for over a month, I made side trips alone. I visited Barcelona and the Prado Museum in Madrid. In Barcelona, people spoke the banned language of Catalan in quiet resistance to the dictator Franco's repression.

I didn't speak either Catalan or Castilian Spanish. My Russian studies remained worthless; my life skills poorly developed, to say the least. I needed to find the youth hostel in Madrid, to find the right track for the train from

Madrid. I needed to eat with the handful of pesetas in my wallet. The solo side trips became rehearsals for finding Sceaux and my mentor alone. Keep my eyes and mind open, don't space out. Learn. Learn fast. The world turned out to be much more complicated than I expected.

---

When we were younger, Dad taught us how the Spanish Civil War was the real start of World War II. Dad's older lefty buddies joined volunteers in Spain to fight for the losing republican side. Democracies, including the US, abandoned the democratically elected government of Spain. The Spanish Fascists, supported by Hitler and Mussolini, triumphed. Fascism worldwide became emboldened. Dad explained fascism, in a word, means "Might makes right."

Stephen argued with him, "That is the way the world works. Survival of the fittest. Nature. Big fish devour little fish."

"That isn't how the world works, Stephen. If that were true, only whales and elephants would exist. Fascism isn't survival of the fittest; it is survival of the cruellest."

## Paris

Mom, Dad, I, and the yellow Volvo crossed the Mediterranean three times by ferry — to or from Haifa, Sicily, Genoa, Tangier, Malaga, Marseilles. The pain in my stomach and fatigue were ever-present. I wasn't in denial. Nothing to be done. The doctor said nothing could be done. Eat this; don't eat that. It didn't seem to matter, or if it did, I didn't notice. Or, I pretended not to notice. My stomach demanded attention, but with no treatment to provide, no medicine, no diet, no supplements: I had only my Buddhist practice, the address from Larry, and the desire to meet my teacher.

In early April 1972, I left my parents in Geneva for a train to Paris. The great adventure, taking a train to Paris. So cool, man on a mission. Sure, others had done this before, but not to meet sensei. By then, I knew how to travel by myself.

Without me, Mom and Dad might even bicker less. Obviously, they loved each other. They seemed so freakishly similar, made for each other, Irene and Ira. And smart. They'd figure out a way to mend what's tearing them apart. I chanted for their happiness.

I didn't speak French and had no contacts. My pockets contained a few US dollars, my passport, and the address from Larry. Dad said he'd send more money.

Arriving at the Paris train station, the glorious Gare de Lyon, I exchanged my dollars for francs, bought a pack of subway tickets. I clutched the now tattered note from Larry, the pirate's treasure map. A huge train and subway map hung on a wall. At the bottom of the map, a word jumped at me, a station named 'Robinson.' That's me. A sign or just another station? Either way, I took hope from seeing my name. Above 'Robinson,' another name — 'Sceaux,' the same impossible word as on Larry's note. Perfect. I will find this place. I can reach Sceaux, the Emerald City, meet the wizard.

---

A train carried me to the Sceaux station. On that station wall hung a map of the town. All right, there's the street. It's near here. Let's find this place. I set off, searching for the address. Everything disoriented me; the street names didn't seem right. I'd find a street sign with a name. But I couldn't figure out which street the sign indicated. The numbers on buildings didn't go in any order I recognized. Spain wasn't this hard. I roamed past large, old, three-storied homes and horse-chestnut and linden trees. Sceaux seemed different from the little I'd seen of Paris. It smelled nice. Not crowded. For an hour or more, I explored clean, winding streets, searching for the address. Pleasant town. Fancy German cars. Carrying my little suitcase, I sweated. I stared at the address on the paper a hundred times and scrutinized street names, baffled.

Defeated, I retraced my steps back to the Sceaux station. Examining the map on the wall now made me frustrated and self-conscious. What's wrong with me? I loved maps and had a good sense of direction. The adventure finished before it began, unless I got assistance.

I showed a station worker the note, the code to the wizard's portal. If only

I could find the portal. The worker pulled me outside and pointed a half block away. All right, that way, certain I'd gone that way.

Another thing, *s'il vous plaît*, I pointed to the word, Sceaux, on the note and the sign above the doors to the station. "How do you say this?"

"Sceaux?" It sounded like "sew", "so." Six letters and three vowels for "so." This language is going to be hard. If only I knew, I'd have taken French in school, instead of Russian. Normal kids took French.

I marched in the direction he'd pointed and there it was, a few steps from the station. I surely passed it. Like the good witch proclaimed to Dorothy, there all along. I rang a buzzer at the gate. A staff member came and let me inside the grounds. Lovely gardens, dark spring green and blooming in the misty early spring afternoon, surrounded the centre.

He and I stood at the entrance to a converted modern home. "I came from America to meet Ikeda-sensei."

The man acted less impressed than in my mind's rehearsal. "Sensei is not here."

"That's okay, I will wait for him." I hadn't thought beyond finding the address in Sceaux. No plan. I mean, once you arrive at the Emerald City, the wizard will take care of everything, right?

In my rehearsal, the wizard took the hero in, amazed by my timely appearance on their doorstep, coming all the way from America. Fed, put to work, even provide a place to sleep.

I couldn't wait at the entrance. I'd return every day if necessary. But I needed to stay somewhere.

―――

The train back to Paris stunk of urine and cigarettes, after the clean spring fragrance of Sceaux. My stomach turned. My mouth tasted bile. All right, let's do this. Find somewhere to stay. I'll wait as long as it takes. I am not alone; I am on my own. This is what I hoped for, to be on my own, seeking sensei. Tomorrow I will go back to Sceaux, find a friendly person who grasps what I am doing in Paris. I came to support. They must prepare for his arrival. I just wanted to help.

That afternoon, I found an apartment on the left bank. Today the room would be illegal — too small for habitation. A former *chambre de bonne*, maid's quarters, had been further divided in two.

The bed lay a single step inside the refitted door. The slope of the roof bisected the room, making standing impossible. Less than eighty square feet, the single room had a half-bed and a paltry table on its last unmatched legs. No chair stood at the table, as a chair couldn't fit between the table and bed.

My choices became lying on the bed or sitting on the bed, using it as my chair for the table. A porthole offered a view of the wall of the building behind. Sixth floor, with no lift, I climbed five floors, then the final set of former servant's stairs. A short timer controlled the dim stairwell light; going completely dark before I got the entire way up or down. Down a flight, I found the shared toilet. Locked, possibly in use. This threatened to be a problem, given my needs. The room took most of my money.

Around this time, new manifestations of Crohn's appeared outside my guts — arthritis, canker sores in my mouth, and psoriasis. The skin around my nose and eyebrows inflamed purply-red, then dried bone white and flaked onto my clothes. On my elbows and knees the skin thinned, becoming raw, bumpy and scaled. The scales inflamed, cracking and bleeding. When I combed my hair, chunks of dry scalp shed, matching the old paint cracking and flaking off the room's walls. At least now nobody could say to me, "it must be in your head. You don't look sick."

## Grappling with Paris

The next morning, I headed out. Forget nothing. I don't want to go back up those six flights of stairs. Take what I need. Be prepared. Be practical, responsible, grow up. This is a strange city, old and cold and stone-grey. I wandered the streets, past magnificent, mysterious buildings, monuments, statues.

About Paris I understood nothing, no weather reports, no way to figure out where to go, the way things work. Brief rain interrupted the day. Be practical; wear the nylon hoodie. Of course, I didn't have weather reports. If I were practical, I wouldn't be in Paris.

The salmon does not understand every rock, every turn in the river on its way home. She returns to spawn, using every ounce of energy, her emaciated body translucent, devoid of fat and flesh. After years in the ocean, she drives back upstream instinctively, to die or find her original natal home. My head didn't comprehend what I longed for, but I grasped instinctively: Paris became where I wanted to be.

The subways proved easy. Follow them along their subterranean paths until I found the right station. The confusion started when I emerged at the station. Which way to go? No road signs resembled those I am used to. No shadows to show north.

I stood at an intersection of roads going several directions, without a clue. Across on the other corner, a guy unfolded an enormous map. And there, on the opposite corner, two people huddled around a map. Well, that's reassuring; everybody's lost.

Underground on the subways, I wasn't lost, safe in the tunnels, round and round. On the train, a guy played accordion up and down the aisle. A kid with him, roughly my age, busked from seat to seat harvesting coins in a braided fibre fedora. A paper handwritten sign hung pinned to his shirt. It may have been their set list, song lyrics, or their tale of woe. The kid doesn't approach me. Maybe my face proclaimed, don't waste time, no money here, I don't belong.

A couple of mornings later, I took the train from the Port-Royal station. The attendant punched my little rectangular ticket stained from my pocket and fingers. He sat alone at the subway entrance, punching everyone's ticket. Clickety-click with his punch tool, over and over. Sad, pinched Gallic face. On my way home, the same guy, same long face, all the long day, hundreds of times, so many passengers, so many clicks. Lonely job among so many. I wanted to say thank you, *merçi*. As I passed him, I said, "Mercy."

He replied, "*Pourquoi?*"

Perhaps he didn't follow me. Or he was sarcastic. Or, he understood English and wondered why, "mercy." *Pourquoi*, why? Yup, that's the question. I am here to meet my teacher. He is coming. I hope someone says when.

Tired, hungry, I should stay in the room until better, gathering my limited strength. Sure, but I can't meet him in my room, can't even find out when he arrives. More than a goal or quest; I breathed to meet him. See his face once, then I can sleep for a long time.

Luckily, along my route to the train station, I found a clean public washroom. And double luck, the washroom had sit toilets, not squat. Timing my trips for when the attendant, "Madame Pipi," cleaned the women's side or took her smoke break, I'd be in and out without paying. At her station she set her kit for duty: rags and buckets and mops and brushes. Users left a *sou* in the dish on her table at the entrance. Not me.

---

I visited the Sceaux centre most every day, volunteering to prepare for sensei's arrival. Whatever they needed, I hoped to pitch in. The place had a large meeting room upstairs and a smaller prayer room below. They allowed visitors to chant in the smaller room. Occasionally, one or two ladies joined me, kneeling on the floor for hours. They wore extra thick socks to protect their ankles. Makes sense. Tomorrow I'll wear two pairs. A tall Japanese lady with wire-rimmed glasses spoke English. We'd grab a break from chanting, go to another room, stretch our frozen legs, sip tea, and chat. She taught a few words of French and Japanese. "You must speak, when Ikeda-sensei arrives."

Some young guys acted polite, but not especially welcoming. They probably wondered what to make of the American kid who didn't seem to do anything but wouldn't go away.

When not at the Sceaux centre, I chanted in my room or drifted the streets alone. One afternoon I shadowed a group of old guys playing *pétanque* in a park. By their clothes, some could have been street sweepers, others university professors. The game remained a mystery. Six or seven men wound over the gravel, throwing metal balls. I dug their body language and dangling cigarettes, the english they spun on the balls. They put it all out: their exaggerated bravado, the tilt of their hats. How were they so unapologetically themselves?

Green spaces and friendly parks stood welcoming from every corner. Meandering through them, I regarded daily life along with the butterflies. Paths in the public gardens and squares lined up with surrounding landmarks and monuments. Someone had their thinking cap on when they designed this place. Cities did not have to resemble Los Angeles. Cities are a choice: how streets are designed, the ways they accommodate people or, in my experience of LA, didn't. I visited free libraries and spent precious francs to visit the Louvre. The parks, streets, monuments beckoned: cities could be beautiful.

## American Express

One of my first mornings, I took the subway across the river to the American Express office at 11 Rue Scribe, near the Opéra Garnier. I wasn't their customer. Teenagers didn't have traveller's cheques or charge cards.

To my surprise, they treated me nicely. I didn't need an account or any special procedure to receive letters or money from Mom and Dad at the office. If something arrived for me, they'd hold it to be claimed. A clerk supplied me with maps, tips on surviving in Paris, information on language classes.

The American Express office became something of a central point for Americans in Paris. Their image reinforced prestige — steamer trunks, alabaster white gloves, and first-class tickets. But 11 Rue Scribe proved more democratic than in their advertising image. Both the fancy well-heeled tourists and the hippies patronized 11 Rue Scribe. Everyone picked up mail, cashed cheques, and shared traveller's tales.

On the steps of the opera house across the street, draft dodgers and runaways sold hashish and played guitars. American and Swedish kids debated revolution and drug runs to Morocco.

## A park in Sceaux

One morning, at the centre in Sceaux, I met up with a few members. One of the young guys said come along and we strolled fifteen minutes to a vast park, the Parc de Sceaux. It had trees blossoming and canals and woods and a chateau. The Sceaux Park impressed as both regal and scaled for individuals. Beautiful. Perfect for a picnic. Or better, I hoped sensei visits this park. The young guys strolled around the park for an hour or so. I envisaged more action or something. Not sure what I expected, but sensei is coming and we are rambling around a park?

One guy, who spoke a little English, mentioned my skin condition. The skin on my hands and elbows, the bridge of my nose and scalp, had thinned, blotchy and peeling. He tried to encourage me, telling of a skin issue he'd had and how his Buddhist practice helped clear it up.

He invited me to a discussion meeting at his apartment on Saturday at 7 p.m. He wrote the address in my pocket note pad. I had trouble reading the address. They wrote numbers and letters differently. He said he lived in Bel-Air. At the park, go right. At least I concluded he said right. Turn right, *droite*, sounded like go straight, *droit*. Anyway, I can figure it out, find the place. There's a Bel-Air in Los Angeles, too. This is great. I am going to get in with these guys, make friends, finally.

## A baguette

That afternoon, on my way back to the apartment, the neighbourhood bakery greeted with the aroma of yeast and warm bread. In line I rehearsed, "*Bonjour, madame. Une baguette, s'il vous plaît.*" The sales person deftly boxed two round layered tidbits for the lady ahead of me. Someday, I'd order whatever those are. And she fetched my loaf and wrapped it in a thin piece of paper, then another lady, the cashier, accepted my money and said *bonne journée*. The exchange and courtesy suggested an old-fashioned charm.

I found a square near the bakery, sat on a bench and contemplated being in Paris for over a week now and still hadn't heard a date for sensei's arrival. A statue of a bearded man with ripped pants and bare feet had a pigeon living on its head, its eyes on my crumbs. You picked the wrong victim, birdie. This loaf stayed mine.

The square felt close, intimate. Foliage of trees and shrubs hung dark-green and wet. I had no idea what the flowers were, but Mom would. Rows of flowers lined the square's walkways, pink and purple and yellow. An old couple with canes sat on the bench across the gravel path, puddles at their feet. On another bench, a young guy wearing a Breton cap and wide colourful tie read a book.

A powder of flour dusted the outside of the loaf. My tongue touched it first, a dry, coarse robe. I carefully bit into the brittle crust, not wanting to spill any. The insides tasted soft and savoury, slightly salty. Each bite differed from the previous; the balance of crust and interior varied as the long loaf disappeared into me. Towards the middle, the pillowy core sprung to my teeth and tongue, while the encasing crust held without crumbling.

Here I sat on a bench, munching my baguette like a character in a book, a man on an adventure. In the book, the square set the stage for an intriguing rendezvous. A furtive, sweat stained agent with acne scars and an uneven mustache delivered a package. Or a woman in sunglasses and trench coat, her high bun tied in a floral bandana, slipped a coded message. Not for me.

I ran solo in my story. My mission. On my own. Fun to be in this square, in my story.

## Different dreams

I finished the baguette in the little square, stomach still unsatisfied. One thing became obvious: I will never comprehend this place and never blend in, but in Paris it didn't seem so crucial that I fit.

Back home, with school, friends, sports, I looked for a space to fit, like a piece from Mom's jigsaw puzzles. If I fit nicely in the puzzle, I had to be sure, so I'd wiggle and twist and turn to make sure I fit. Twisting until the cardboard edges of the piece frayed and I mismatched again.

Here in Paris, fitting in wasn't going to happen. I needed to figure out how I could help with sensei's visit and stayed fed and housed until whenever he arrived. I'd never been so alone. Had I someone to talk to, how could they understand what I was doing?

Whoever built this beautiful city and this square figured out how to make their city a little more beautiful. And those who lived here now, amongst all this beauty, did their bit too.

Look at how they carefully dress, even on the train, and the way they arranged flowers out on those thin balconies, making room for a touch of colour and joy. Yesterday I wandered up to the river and found some people watching a dance. I joined the audience. A dozen couples and families danced to a woman playing a violin and another person on a cello. They didn't appear to be a performance, just folks getting outside to celebrate spring.

Sometimes the French came across as arrogant, or possibly I misinterpreted their shyness. They certainly didn't seem to worry who they were. Sure, the train held long faces, the same as buses in LA. And most of those on the train or streets looked poorer than in LA. But they seemed better at being poor, if that makes any sense. Not saying they became resigned to poverty, just better at it. In the States, we weren't as good at being poor, even though we had lots of poor people. Maybe it's the whole American Dream thing, expecting that everybody should acquire everything. Probably Parisians had different dreams. For me, today, here on this bench, my dreams felt fine.

To me, life in the States drove forward relentlessly, without memory or self-reflection, without the beauty of context. In *Notes of a Native Son*, James Baldwin wrote, "Perhaps it now occurs to him that in this need to establish himself in relation to his past, he is most American, that this depth-less alienation from oneself and one's people is, in sum, the American experience."[42]

Say what you will about Paris; it has depth. I rambled the streets and public spaces, captivated by history and culture. The signs on the imposing buildings remained meaningless, incomprehensible. I knew nothing of who built them or when, or the history of this king or that revolution. But a living, modern city bustled through these ancient roads. The city wasn't a museum; I observed vibrant life inside its monuments and boulevards and gardens alike.

As everywhere, regular folk struggled to survive. But within that struggle, they made daily living more beautiful, refined. I approached its labyrinth naïvely, receptively. Paris said it's okay to not comprehend, to be an outsider. Let go of preconceptions and expectations and allow myself to be transformed.

The Spanish writer Carlos Ruiz Zafón: "Paris is the only city in the world where starving to death is still considered an art."[43] Lonely, tired, hungry, sick, I became the protagonist of my story set in the city's mystery.

## The bakery

Francs disappeared, and I had no idea how long my thinning supply needed to last. The room cost sixty or seventy francs a week. Roughly $15. Larry said sensei would arrive in April, but mid-April came and went and nobody at the Sceaux centre knew a date.

Once a day, I had my ritual at the bakery. Arriving, a moment of hesitation at the forest green door. The lever handle looked like a turn-and-push, but the door pulled out to the street. When I forgot and pushed, the frame and glass and hanging *ouvert* sign rattled drawing curious, and, I imagined, disapproving, eyes in my direction. The slight step up inside the entrance invited me to trip onto the polished tile floor. Looking up, the ceiling was hammered metal. Groovy. Surviving the entrance, the aromas of bread, sugar, and pastry welcomed me. The display counters overflowed with mysterious, unpronounceable delights. Against the far wall baskets filled with different breads. But I was there for one thing, my daily baguette.

A sales lady took my order, another wrapping, even a third to take money; bread for everybody forever. The exchange always concluded with a sunny *bonne journée*. The government set the price of baguettes. Memory says 75 centimes for a loaf, around 15 US cents. The bakery always had a brief line, a couple of customers in front and behind me. In my imagination, the line stretched back in time; if I'd been in the bakery a hundred years prior, a few customers in front, a handful behind me. They both over-complicated and charmed with a simple transaction worth a few cents. But the daily experience comforted. I participated in an age-old flow of nourishing bread, consuming a single loaf a day. Not enough.

## Lost in Bel-Air

That Saturday evening, I set off to meet the guys I'd met at the park in Sceaux. Exiting the #6 subway at the old brick Bel-Air station. I pulled my notepad from my back pocket. Rain soaked the pad, smearing the guy's address. Well, I can figure this out: the paper had said number something on rue something, turn right at the park, or go straight. No park outside the station. I followed the station road to a major intersection where four or five streets crossed. Every other crossing in Paris looked similar and nothing looked distinguishing. I meandered around, hoping for a sign, or the guy to pop up looking for me, or find the park, or something.

I hadn't eaten since the morning. My guts cramped. With the clouds, dusk came. Not only did I miss the rendezvous, but now I'd forgotten how to get back to the subway. The rain fell hard.

An underpass ran under an old train line, overgrown vegetation and broken, twisted steel and concrete. I'd wait under its shelter for the rain to halt. A bearded man propped against the wall cradled a bottle. The dank underpass stunk of vomit and piss and stale wine. And cheap tobacco smoke. At the other end, two silhouetted figures smoked. Not the place to test the kindness of Parisians. I fled, panicking that I wouldn't find my way back to the flat. Visions of a phone call from the American embassy. "Doctor and Mrs. Robinson, I am afraid we have bad news." I wouldn't make friends, wouldn't meet my mentor, everything wasted.

It took a couple of hours, but I made my way across the Seine River and found the apartment. I trudged up the dark apartment stairs, my stomach empty, my guts burning, humiliated at failing to meet the guys. Exhausted and famished, I pulled off my wet clothes, collapsed on the bed, and slept eighteen hours.

## Lunch at the Sorbonne

When I woke late Sunday afternoon, I stayed in, chanting and sleeping more. Uncertain whether just tired and hungry or something more serious, I sat up and chanted. I blew it with those guys; I stood them up, flaked, blowing my shot at connection. Couldn't even find an address, show up on time. And here I'd imagined myself as the great helper. I blew it.

What if I was sick, I mean, sick-sick? The concierge lady might have offered aid if I figure out how to tell her I need a doctor. That would ruin everything, go to the hospital, never meet Ikeda. After everything, to blow it. I drifted back to sleep.

Monday, forty-eight hours since I had eaten, I ventured out, carrying a binder and a few books. I snuck into the Sorbonne University student lunch hall. Memories of the 1968 student revolution were still fresh, so soldiers guarded the universities. Vigilant soldiers with serious rifles and serious expressions stood at the school entrances. With the props under my arm and a studious expression, I passed the soldiers into the ancient university.

A lunch ticket cost a couple of francs. I ate and ate alone, elbow to elbow amongst hundreds of real students on long tables in the enormous student mess. My lonely stomach filled with beans and sausage and fatty stew ladled from caldrons. Belly stuffed, I grabbed slices of bread from the common baskets and crammed my jacket pockets full. They even had carafes of wine on the communal tables.

With a solid meal and the spare bread in my pockets, I'd survive. Still, after three weeks, I required money and a cheaper place to sleep. I headed back to the American Express office. The same diligent clerk who'd assisted previously looked after me. I explained my predicament — I expected money any day, but wasn't sure how much; I might be staying another few weeks.

Her finger slid across a page in a binder. She phoned a hostel on the right bank for Asian and African students. A bunk cost five francs a night, a little over a dollar; more for a blanket and sheet. They had a space.

One last trip to the apartment to pick up my suitcase and say *au revoir* to the concierge. The slightest shrug of her shoulders and bewildered look conveyed she wasn't sorry I was leaving; she'd never figured out why I'd come.

## Hostel for Asian and African students

Not Asian, African, or a student, I stayed in the hostel's dorm with renegades, misfits, and students from Syria, Vietnam, Cameroon, the Congo. The gates locked at 10. If I returned from Sceaux after 10, no bunk that night.

I had the top of a bare metal bunk in a room with three other guys, two Africans and one Arab. Each had a story, one running away, another kicked out of their country, and the third, an amicable man from Congo going to university. They weren't phony or posturing, without any need to impress. I enjoyed wonderful conversations with the guys at the hostel, the ones who spoke English. Their unique perspectives on travel and politics opened my eyes, challenging my assumptions. Each story had worth.

I don't remember any women at the hostel; they may have had their own space.

---

For a couple of hours, we hung out in the hostel's common room. The guy from the Congo, the student, probed, "Why are you here?" His bright, round face looked concerned.

"I am waiting for my teacher. He is coming from Japan to teach about peace and Nam-myoho-renge-kyo."

"Do you miss your family?" He missed his, sharing stories of his home. On the wall behind his bunk, he'd taped pictures of siblings and endless cousins and aunts back home. He became the first in his sprawling family to leave home for school in France.

I missed regular dinners and my books and a bed with a pillow, but did I miss my family? I remained sick and lonely. But homesick? He happily spoke about his family in the Congo, so I inquired about growing up in a close family you'd miss. But he still had questions for me, "You left home in America to come to France to meet your teacher from Japan?"

Hadn't considered it that way. "Hard to explain. He is my life's teacher and I've never met him. He's very important to me."

Hanging with my dorm-mates in the hostel felt part of a grand flow of humanity. Here I stayed among strangers, outlaws and outcasts and students who roamed the same ancient streets. Still, I didn't belong here, in this hostel for Asian and African students. For all the allure of this fascinating city, I didn't belong in Paris, either.

That night, in my metal upper bunk, the guy from the Congo snoring beneath me, I reflected, am I homesick? It might be cool if the family were here. Stephen would embrace the freedom to be himself. Peter, too, might jive; I hear the French are crazy for jazz. Mom would love the art and gardens. Dad and I would discuss urban design, housing, and transport. We'd talk politics. Be happy, bicker less.

## The boulevard

The Arab from our room befriended me. He came from Syria, via Shatalova, USSR. The Soviets were after him, he explained, for deserting their Air Force training program. For a guy claiming to be on the run, he showed none of the nerves of a hustler or fugitive.

One afternoon he bought me coffee on the Boulevard Saint-Michel. By now I expected the daily overcast skies, interrupted by warm sun, then short bursts of rain. We sat side-by-side in the diffuse April light at a round metal bistro table. We discussed philosophy and Buddhism, art and socialism, the stuff you are supposed to discuss on the boulevard.

A clopping pulled my attention to the crowded back-and-forth on the boulevard. Paris criss-crossed by our seats: cars, buses, bikes, men wearing cravats and wide ties and women walking their pups. The clopping persisted. Undisturbed by the bustle, a work-horse pulled a cart past our café, its hooves thick as a tree, eyes soft with purpose, step by steady step.

"Drink slowly," my relaxed Arab friend-on-the-run taught, "we are going to be here for the afternoon. A single cup will do. Have you been to the Louvre?"

We lifted our tiny cups of coffee to our lips pretending to sip, the deep nutty aroma filled my nose. "When I first got here."

"So much to see. So much beauty. A single visit is not enough. How do you call her? *La Joconde* . . . the Madonna . . . Mona Lisa? Ah, she deserves at least a whole day to be with her . . . she is so . . ." He says something in Arabic, coming from the back of his throat, from below his throat, from his belly. Then, in English, each syllable individually, "magnificent." His voice trails. Wow, having coffee outside a Paris café with a fugitive who is in love with a lady in a painting.

I've seen those old-timey sepia photographs of the fashionable folk on the boulevard. They're sitting at the round tables, elegantly dressed, writing books or falling in love. Who are those people? What sort of people are they, so happy?

For a few hours one afternoon in 1972, I sat where the beautiful people sat. For a few hours, I forgot the cramps, my burning skin. On my quest. I really was in Paris.

## The Ikedas arrive, Friday, 28 April

And a quest I was on. Back to Sceaux. At the centre, I met another man, a doctor, the leader of the European Soka Gakkai. Balding, he wore a snazzy bowtie and a warm, open face.

When I told him I wanted to meet Ikeda-sensei, he beamed.

"*Formidable*! I heard a young American came here, wanting to aid us. Splendid." I preferred the doctor, nicer than the first man.

I inquired when sensei would arrive. "We don't know yet. He is going to London to meet the historian Arnold Toynbee. We are waiting for the schedule." The doctor introduced me to other French young men. Together we moved furniture and desks to create an office, built a small stage in the centre's garden, among other tasks. In my stumbling, clumsy way, I tried to assist the French members prepare for sensei's arrival. Probably I caused more trouble than support.

Toward the end of April, I made a daily trek to the American Express office, lining up at the clerk's window. I waited for money from Dad while waiting for sensei to arrive.

---

On April 27th, I assisted an advance staff member from Japan preparing arrival documents. Ikeda and his wife, Kaneko, were en route. The French members readied the large room upstairs for a gathering. The next day, one of the young men directed me to the same small downstairs prayer room where I'd chanted long hours. I waited in the small room for the last time, initially alone, then others joined me. About eight of us chanted together, excited and nervous, inside a little cloud of sandalwood incense smoke.

After the gathering upstairs, sensei and Mrs. Ikeda came down to the little room. I stood to greet them. "Welcome to Paris." In his early forties, the short Japanese man in a yellow sweater shook my hand. He looked so happy to be there, right where he was, beaming, in the moment, present. As if he were welcoming me. Mrs. Ikeda also smiled, her eyes observant, absorbing everything. The couple moved together in tandem, as though in a graceful dance.

My quest was fulfilled.

## One week in Sceaux

I spent another week in the amazing City of Lights, attending daily prayer and other events with Daisaku and Kaneko Ikeda. His secretary assigned me various tasks. I ran errands, delivered messages, organized books and boxes of this and that. I worked wholeheartedly to help him. Hundreds of members, friends and well-wishers gathered from around Europe and Africa. Some brought small gifts, postcards, or souvenirs from their country. Daisaku and Mrs. Ikeda responded with gifts they'd brought — prayer beads, scarves, books.

The couple tirelessly encouraged members and non-members, children and dignitaries. One morning after prayers, sensei patiently taught two hundred members and guests how to take part in the Japanese tea ceremony. He and Kaneko hosted a garden party on the centre's grounds and planted a cedar tree.

Nothing transcendent happened that week. Ikeda performed no magic tricks. He did what Mom and Dad hoped to do themselves — practical, daily steps for peace. Mom and Dad dearly hoped that I would carry on their efforts for peace, humanity, justice. I wanted to reply to their hopes. Something inside registered. I knew. This week defined who I would become — not my disease, not my family, not my pervasive angst.

On May 3, Daisaku and Kaneko attended a prayer meeting for the attainment of world peace. He told those who gathered, "Polish your character to its highest level. Carry out the mission that you were born for and enable your whole family to live together in happiness. Pursuing this goal, many hardships may confront you, but always making your faith as your prime point, I would like for you to overcome these."[44]

These words arrived third hand, delivered in Japanese, translated to French, then roughly relayed to me later. Despite the indirect delivery, I received their simple message with my guts. My needy, fractured family deserved better. I had to polish my character and support us to come together. The words drove into me, shaking me.

That drizzling evening, outside the Sceaux centre, he waited for his wife and a car to take them to dinner. The helpful bow-tied doctor with him translated as we exchanged a few words. The light rain was a hint of storms to come. When those storms raged, I wanted to be with him, not physically, but whatever way I could. I pictured myself holding an umbrella over his head.

That week, I committed. Ikeda was working to transform the troubled destiny of humanity. Towards that end, he forged ties with like-minded people and groups worldwide. I would do everything in my ability to support him and be part of that arduous effort. I didn't want to be his student, fan, or a follower. If I and my family had the remotest chance for happiness, I must, as he'd said, face and overcome my difficulties. In my mind, my youthful, awkward passion, I'd received a mandate, like a medieval esquire, without ceremony or oath, accepting a sacred accolade. Nobody had to recognize my resolve; Ikeda needn't know. My idealism turned to a quiet sense of purpose, though I had no practical idea what to do.

At the end of the week, Daisaku and Kaneko left for London. Money from Dad arrived at the American Express office. I left Paris, met up with Mom and Dad in Scandinavia, and soon returned to LA alone.

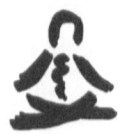

# Courage

Darkness
Source of silent, seminal energy,

Dawn
lying at the pale intersection of purpose and resignation,

Stretch
reaching to the bridges and strains

Open
tiny portals of creation,

Choices
built on anxiety or excavated with hope,

Courage
not the absence of fear,

Courage
not the absence of caution,

Courage is action
it ain't about your head or heart or feelings.

The mentor
pushing his pen forward again today,

The student
what will you push forward today?

Night
rest and dream of tomorrow's pivotal struggle.

# Siddhartha's Fall

### Nairañjanā River, Kingdom of Magadha, 445 BCE

SIDDHARTHA HIT BOTTOM. To solve the riddle of the self, he came to the brink of destroying himself. He accompanied five ascetics who endeavoured to control the self through self-abuse. Together with the five, he engaged in extreme self denial and mortification. He stood on a single leg for hours, consumed only bird droppings, and denied himself sleep for days. He meditated to subdue his mind, repudiate his doubts and angst. His body drained, his mind plunged into turmoil. Emaciated, he undoubtedly suffered permanent internal damage.

Before his final collapse, instead of continuing to self-destruct, he stopped. This is not working. He set out to free, not destroy himself. Life is worth more. Find another way.

### Memories of a rose-apple tree

He stumbled along the banks above the Nairañjanā. Fading now, a childhood memory broke through his delirium. He remembered sitting under the shade of a spreading rose-apple tree watching his father supervise work in the fields. The child Siddhartha, safe and secluded, entered a pleasant, contemplative state. His bottom on the ground, his hands combed through the grass. Happily focused on his setting and the moment, the child sat within the glow and the warm air on his face and arms, under the sunshine dappled leaves. The sun warmed little Siddhartha. The grass tickled and comforted his bottom. His father's orders to the workers, the buzz of insects, the wind rustling the leaves, reached his ears.

The thirty-four-year-old Siddhartha stood, legs shaky, starved and defeated, on the edge of death. He bent and with gaunt, sunken eyes, stared at the grass by the riverbank. His emaciated frame leaned towards the ground. He reached, tottering, as if the child sat in his view, as if the child were with him by the Nairañjanā, sitting in rapture under a rose-apple tree.

Siddhartha stayed with the memory. His studies, his questioning, his self-abuse converged on this moment. Siddhartha realized the pointlessness of denying his body, rejecting his own mind. Denying the common denies the divine, for the divine lies only within the common.

But he could do nothing. Weakened, near death, too late. As he opened to possibilities, his body gave out. He stumbled, foundering. He grasped for a branch or rock, anything to balance.

Siddhartha's legs failed. He toppled, spent, swallowed by darkness.

# My Fall

> I went astray from the straight road
> and woke to find myself alone in a dark wood.
> How shall I say what wood that was!
> I never saw so drear, so rank,
> so arduous a wilderness!
> Its very memory gives a shape to fear.[45]
>
> Dante Alighieri

## Expectations meet reality, Los Angeles, May 1972

BACK FROM EUROPE, ALONE, I expected my life to take off, dreaming of a future assisting my mentor and helping others. For the first time, I'd found a place to fit, a place I wanted to fit, sharing Ikeda's vision of personal growth, contributing to my family and our anguished world. My vision for what I could do, who I was with Crohn's or without, expanded. My quest fulfilled, I imagined I'd achieved something. Wrong. Fulfilling life's purpose took more effort than a few weeks of wandering around Europe.

In the beginning, I got lucky. My original plane ticket had been from LA to Tel Aviv, return. But I returned from Oslo, a lower fare. Money remained on the ticket. The helpful lady at the Pan Am office in LA refunded a couple of hundred dollars. Stephen had a car to loan, a 1963 VW beetle. A car and money to start off.

Over the next two years, my health and life deteriorated. I entered university, unequipped financially and unprepared for the workload. Borrowing the money, I flew to Japan to see my mentor again and returned to a mailbox of unpaid bills and an eviction notice. That night, my roommate and I shared a duty-free brandy bottle mixed with Tang.

To survive, I drove courier, ruining the VW and accumulating over seventy unpaid parking and traffic tickets. The pain in my stomach became unremitting, my belly hot to the touch. I drove with my pants belt undone and passed out twice behind the wheel.

As I became sicker, it became harder and harder to chant consistently and next to impossible in hospital. I lost external supports, and I forgot to look within. Failing to live up to my own values increased my shame and defensiveness. My mentor said, polish my character, develop myself so my family could be harmonious. Instead, I clung to ever weakening strands of my specialness. So different, nobody gets me. Nobody notices my invisible pain. No one can help. As I suffered more and more loss, I had few inner resources to summon.

By 1974, I hung at the edge of death: septic, bowels perforated and disintegrating. My roommate carried me into the emergency room. The emergency doctors contacted Dr. Goldberg. They booked a surgeon and room to operate, my first emergency surgery. The surgeon removed roughly a third of my intestine.

In the recovery room, Goldberg explained a large section of both the large and small bowel had deteriorated to the point it became "no longer viable. Your bowel ruptured. This takes time. We aren't sure how you survived without functioning guts." Three hundred fifty years earlier, Dr. Fabry stood in front of the body of a dead teen and wondered the same.

A week after the surgery, still in pain and drowsy with morphine, I tried to take a shower. Struggling with my IV pole, I maneuvered into the washroom. Something wet streamed down my abdomen and legs. Opening the hospital gown, greenish white goo issued from my belly onto the tiled shower floor. I heard Dr. Goldberg calling me.

I scream in reply from the shower, "You bastard, you cut me. My guts are coming out."

Goldberg stuck his head into the washroom. "Keith, you can't speak to me that way." Legs shaking, I turned to him. Now he saw. "I'll fetch the surgeon. That isn't your guts. Let's get you into bed."

My wound had become infected. The surgeon tore off the tape holding the incision and cleaned the wound. Later, a nurse demonstrated how to clean myself using 4X4 cotton pads, sanitising alcohol in a bottle, and a stinky blood-red liquid. To avoid further infection, they didn't re-close me. This decision led to four decades of physical and emotional trauma.

## The hole, 1974–2014

They left the incision open to heal naturally. Over years, the internal plastic sutures worked their way to the surface, causing minor infections. Each suture had to be cut and pulled out. Dozens of them, a couple at a time. Little off-white and puce-red pus and blood volcanoes surfaced through my belly, staining my shirt. The stain's the cue: another internal suture started coming out. Once in a while, I tried to remove them myself. Dumb. More infections, more mess.

As a result, the muscle wall never healed, causing a permanent hernia that deteriorated from bad to worse. I moved back to Canada and eventually became certified by the International Sommelier Guild. The guild educates sommeliers in beverage service and knowledge. My job included carrying wine cases off trucks, up and down restaurant cellar stairs. Being a sommelier is 90% glamorous, 10% grunt labour. The hernia hole grew.

More emergency surgeries for blocked bowels further deteriorated the muscle wall. Doctors tried surgeries several times to repair the mess. They operated for Crohn's. They operated for the hernias caused by operating for Crohn's. Hernias, tears in muscle walls, are dangerous because a loop of bowel might get snared in the tear, squeezed, strangled, and burst. Untreated people die. Not me. My hernia became so huge a fist fit inside it. Lengths of bowel slid in and out, with no danger strangling. How to get through my day with a fist-sized hole in my stomach wall is less clear.

They inserted fabric mesh inside my abdomen. The mesh tore and failed. They tried plastic wire nettings. Failed. They wrapped me in girdles to wear under my shirt. These made me hot and sweaty and their velcro fasteners popped open at the guaranteed most embarrassing times. Surgeries for Crohn's opened me. Surgeries for the hernia tried to seal me closed. Eleven total. Throughout, my stomach bulged even with girdles. Coworkers made fun of it. It looked, um, distended. This helped me learn empathy for others with visible oddities.

In 2014, forty years after the first hole that had never closed, a brilliant young surgeon from Ethiopia opened me. He dug out the tattered, decomposing remains of the old nettings, now inter-grown with fat and muscle. He installed a numbered device made of pork collagen to replace the failed fabric and plastic nets. So far, the sheet-like porcine biomesh implant has kept insides in and outsides out. He tells me it was the most demanding surgery he's ever performed, eleven hours over me. Getting the ten thousand dollar surgical implant took a special procurement from the Health Ministry. And a pig.

## Another Keith, Kaiser Permanente Hospital, Los Angeles

Back in 1974, after my first surgery, Dr. Goldberg told me of another kid with Crohn's in the same hospital. His name, coincidentally, was Keith, Keith White. Goldberg said Keith's condition was severe and life threatening. Unlike me, he probably would not go home. "He's not my patient, but they've asked me to consult, because of the similarities with your case." Once I became mobile, the doctor gave me the kid's room number, hoping I might encourage him. I think Goldberg also wanted me to realize I wasn't alone.

The nurse injected a morphine shot in my butt. She cleaned my dressing and adjusted my IV, using a stopwatch to calculate drip time. She made a note on my patient record card with a fat ball-point pen that held black, blue, and red ink, a different colour for each nursing shift. Ready to go, tied to my IV pole, I headed out, looking for a room with a kid with Crohn's named Keith.

I found his private room. Two Keiths in a room. Both in hospital gowns. Me, holding on to my IV pole for stability. Him, attached to drains and feeding tubes, and monitors and hospital stuff. A skinny, dark-haired kid in a hospital bed stared up, eyes weak. Prostrate. Around my age.

He concentrated. "Who are you? What are you doing here?"

I examined his IV drip, the feeding tube, and the heart monitor, forced out a few words: "Keith, what have they done to you?" Acting casual and curious but actually terrified. A few years prior, my doctor said my case was rare and now here's another kid my age, with my name. Like a twin. I stood, unsure, staring down at him. Staring at each other. Mirrors. Surgically cracked mirrors. As if we peered into each other's futures, futures colliding. Two broken bellies. Mine, maybe healing. His, probably not.

Don't consider that; encourage him; offer hope. Kind of hard to encourage when my mouth is so dry, lips trembling, hand gripping the IV pole until my knuckles whiten. He might be me. I wanted to bolt. Holding my breath, I froze, terrified for us both. That bastard doctor sent me. The inflamed skin around my IV port screamed to be scratched. Keith told me he'd been sick for a few years. Nobody knew what was wrong.

"About a year ago, they operated. They tried to resect as little of the small intestine as possible; just remove the damaged part and reconnect the healthy gut. Remove as little as possible. But it didn't get better. It came back and got worse in the same place where they sliced. So, they operated again. They found the inflammation had spread from the place where they operated the first time. And that kept happening. I never had time to recover from one surgery before I needed another. Each time in the exact place they cut before."

I didn't want him to suffer like that. But he did. No use being there. I couldn't help. No one could help. There he lay, right in front of me, inches away. His damaged guts lay inches away, right there. I almost saw them through his robe and what remained of thin skin and scar. No force on Earth existed to rescue him.

Keith said, "I don't care anymore. I want to go home." My eyes drifted. Flowers, a card on a table. Home. He came from somewhere. Had loved ones who wanted him to recover. Wanted him to return home. Wanted him to not suffer.

I visited Keith White four or five times. Over the previous year, he had been through nine major surgeries, each time a further section of bowel removed. Mostly, I stood and listened to his story. Sedated, he'd fade in and out.

During one visit, he showed me his stomach, a mass of scar tissue. Nine surgeries. One year. Nine slices. Nine scarred Vs. Emaciated, his ribs protruded. My future lay there fed through a tube, carved and carved again.

I stayed in hospital for around six months, dealing with the infection and other complications and recovering. During that time, the courier company fired me. My roommate got engaged, and I hadn't paid rent. So he told me not to return. Where should he send my stuff?

Dad had accepted a position at a university in Canada. He and Mom sold the Los Feliz house. They had split up, then got back together, renting an apartment in Long Beach, near Los Angeles. They travelled back and forth to Calgary. For a few months, they let me stay in Long Beach to recuperate.

The day of my discharge, I visited Keith White for the last time. He'd further declined, barely conscious. Not to disturb him, I left a note on his side table and, in a whisper, chanted three times. The hospital sent me off with gauze, packing squares, and smelly red goop to keep my open surgical wound uninfected.

## Broken, 1974–1975

Out of the hospital, I recovered at my parents in Long Beach. One part of me said, I'm fixed. Bullshit, fooling myself, badly. I'm recovering from surgery, this incident, not recovering from the disease, just from this incident. Nineteen years old, I lay on my back, cleaning the wound. So much to go wrong.

My life headed down the tubes. My parents moved to Calgary, and I was on my own again. The unpaid traffic tickets caught up with me. Twice the police came and took me to jail. The bank repossessed my car. The state revoked my driver's license. My girlfriend dumped me.

Desperate, I stole stereos off a loading dock to sell and stole money from friends.

The embers of my quest still smouldered. But in my despair, when I most needed my practice, I neglected it. I never lost complete touch with my practice, my ideals, or my sense of connection to Ikeda. But I'd lost the ability to pursue it. My shame deepened.

I longed for what I'd lost: to turn back the clock, deserve my girlfriend back, to have done so many things differently. I didn't want to live with Crohn's. Another impossible longing. If only I didn't have CD, if only I became normal. Not be tired all the time. Finish school. Make a difference. Hail the revolution.

Still, I wanted to live a life of purpose, to align my life with my teacher's purpose. By 1975, I was floundering in that challenge, in a downward spiral of loss and shame and regret. Whatever I dreamt of doing, being a thief wasn't on my list. Thieving I did.

No, I didn't forget my Buddhist practice; I forgot to use it. I forgot to turn the energy of my longings toward developing myself. As I lost one thing, then another, the walls closed in, my life and faith choices narrowed. In the end, I forgot about my growth and developing my character. I wasn't able to support my parents or even feed myself. My quest lay buried under the ash of poor decisions. And I loathed myself for that. So smart; seen and done so much. So clever. I knew nothing. I was a mess.

Don't blame Crohn's or my childhood or anyone for my implosion. I got there alone. The worst proved not what happened to me, or even anything I'd done. I'd abandoned the values my parents instilled in me and my mentor's trust.

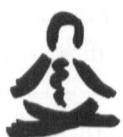

# "Yo-chan, we will meet again."

## Leaving Aino Village, 1971

THROUGHOUT MY SCHOOL YEARS, I kept in mind sensei's hope for young people to work for peace on a grand world stage. Even as a child, I dreamt of becoming a capable person contributing to a peaceful society. But I did not know how to make it happen. All I knew was, staying in Aino Village would not make it happen.

Moving to a big city would be a step toward learning about the world and leaving Japan behind. The Soka Gakkai newspaper showed pictures of thousands of enthusiastic members at events in large cities. After high school, I worked for a home products company in Osaka for three years, saving every yen to move overseas. The Netherlands was famous for flowers, so I dreamed of going to Holland. Yes, I was that naïve.

In those days, as today, tens of thousands of Osakans practised with Soka Gakkai. Living in Osaka, I saw how Soka Gakkai contributed to regular people's lives, but on a scale I'd only imagined.

## Women mentors of Osaka

One time I attended a Soka Gakkai rally of thousands of young women members. Coming from tiny Aino, I'd never experienced youthful dedication and passion on such a scale. My eyes opened and my mind exploded in awe. Powerful young women united for peace. Everyone worked side-by-side, without gossiping or comparing or speaking from jealousy. This movement is happening. World peace is possible.

I also attended smaller, local discussion meetings. One lady held gatherings in her rambling home. Her large, old-fashioned house stood out in our crowded community of apartment blocks and dormitories. I loved the gatherings at her place, meeting Osakans, young and old. Twenty-five or more of us packed into her living room. Back home, I attended meetings with Mom and Dad. But here in Osaka, on my own, I found a new family.

She also used her house for classes in flower arrangement and the tea ceremony. My company had a budget for personal development and she gave me a discount for her classes. From her, I gained skills in traditional arts that I've used to this day.

One time, she gave me a ticket to a classical *Noh* theatre performance in Kyoto. She even gave me tips on dress and behaviour. To attend the traditional drama, dance, and music theatre was a once in a lifetime opportunity. She also took me to major flower arranging and tea ceremony events. "Yoshiko, don't miss any opportunity to learn. Seize each chance and do your best. Never forget to represent our movement well."

Another lady who came to the local gatherings also became a mentor. Dr. Nishi was a dentist, a profession in those days reserved for men. Women could only be dental assistants, receptionists, or hygienists. To pursue her profession, she faced and overcame tremendous hindrances.

Dr. Nishi dressed in tailored silk men's suits and ties, her hair slicked back like a man's. Without make-up, wearing men's spectacles, she looked like a successful Italian financier. What a beautiful woman, always positive and cheerful. She never frowned or said a harsh word. Dr. Nishi taught me to live with pride, with dignity and confidence and never apologize for being myself. She served me tea and delicious pastries in her exquisitely furnished apartment. Later, I ended up in the dental industry.

Another senior member gave me care in faith, Ms. Izumi, a stunning, freckled flight attendant. Her airline had a well-appointed staff dormitory next door to my company's simple facility.

In my company's dorm, I shared a room with two other girls. Difficult to chant without disturbing my roommates, I waited until they slept and recited the sutra in a whisper. Sometimes I snuck next door. Ms. Izumi had her own room, and we chanted together. Her colleagues were friendly, although they didn't join us in prayers.

For my nineteenth birthday, Ms. Izumi treated me to Osaka's finest French restaurant. On my way home from the train station, I walked by that restaurant, but never imagined eating anywhere so special. Then we entered side by side; me the proud, nervous acolyte. I wore a new one piece black dress with a choker. Ms. Izumi dressed stylish as ever, her perfect proportions in a pastel cream turtleneck with pearl necklace. We stepped into the entrance surrounded by greenery and fresh flowers and up two steps to the dining area. Other customers and staff are blotted from my memory. Only this beautiful teacher who confidently and oh so casually brought me to my first French restaurant.

She ordered a seafood gratin and *sole meunière* with white wine for me. Fish. That evening, I ate and enjoyed fish. Surrounded by white napkins and tablecloths and beautiful china, I felt so fancy.

Hers was a sad story, as a mistress to a wealthy married business executive. Like me, she came from a small coastal town. "Yoshiko," she'd declare, "take pride in who you are. You must achieve every single one of your dreams." Never accept poor treatment; never accept second best. She had to find a way forward from her dead-end relationship. Above all, her intelligence, elegant manner, and our Buddhist practice would guide her.

My dormitory did not include a bath or shower, so I used a public bathhouse four blocks away. Usually my two dormmates and I went together. It was fun bathing together and safer too. We also travelled together to work, when we could. Our route to the office passed a small park where a flasher lurked. Every morning, he exposed himself to women on their daily way. So, we three stuck together, closely trailing random male pedestrians for cover.

---

One rainy night, however, I headed home from the bath late and alone on the empty street. A man followed me. I hurried. He walked faster. I ran, gripping my plastic pail with clothes and toiletries; he ran faster. My place was too far; I could not make it safely, so I ran up the stairs to the airline's side. There he was, at the bottom of the stairs, looking up at me.

"Ms. Izumi, help!"

Fortunately, they hadn't locked the door to their dormitory. My friend took me into the common room. She and four or five other flight attendants surrounded me, calmed me down, then fed me. From alone and terrified to embraced by caring, strong women, doting over and indulging me.

These confident, worldly women taught me so much. Soka Gakkai brought us together, so I appreciate them and our organisation. All over the world, moving to big cities can crush country girls. The heartless machine of modern living often destroyed precious young lives.

This country minnow swam in Osaka's big pond. Instead of drowning me, the city nurtured every aspect of my life. My vision of life, the organisation, and our goal of peace expanded.

While in Osaka, I visited Kyoto and its museums many times. I stood in front of paintings by Monet and Renoir. The paintings filled my eyes and embraced my heart. Love at first sight. Such beauty. Picasso took longer, demanded I work harder, but over time, he seduced me too. I came to Osaka to learn more about the world, and every day held valuable lessons.

I took English classes and spoke to agencies and anyone with information about moving abroad. The owner of the English school, a Canadian guy, taught the advanced classes. I didn't qualify for his class. But one day, he came to our beginner's class and spoke to us about Canada, its free, natural beauty. He said if you go fishing in Canada in lakes, rivers, or the oceans, you don't need bait. Just throw in a hook on a line and pull out a fish. Despite my complete lack of interest in fish or fishing, the story stuck in my mind.

Around that time, a girl from Aino moved to Canada to live with her uncle and aunt in Calgary. Pauline was younger than me, so we didn't play together. Her big sister Harumi was the middle of us three crows, roaming the fields and woods of Mount Daisen.

## Canada, 1974

Despite the contacts I made in Osaka, Pauline remained my only solid connection with the world outside Japan. And so, after turning twenty-one, I left Japan for Canada, alone. I wrote three goals for my new life: help spread Nichiren Buddhism, contribute to Canadian society, and build a harmonious family.

The first week, I stayed with Pauline and her aunt and uncle. Pauline entered high school by this time and they both worked, so I took care of myself. Her aunt made me sandwiches for my lunch. I set up a bank account, walked to the post office, and learned how to ride the bus.

At the end of the week, I left Pauline's and worked in the beautiful home of a prominent family. The Cohen family started with nothing. Five brothers and one cousin in Winnipeg could only afford a single suit between them. If one boy had a business meeting, he would wear the suit. They built an electronics empire across Canada.

Many years later, after Keith and I were married, we drove past the old Jewish Funeral Home on Seventeenth Avenue. One man, dressed in an immaculately tailored suit and carrying a plastic bag, roamed alone back and forth across the empty parking lot. My old boss, Harry Cohen, picked litter off the pavement, cleaning after others. Keith said, "Harry Cohen could hire a hundred janitors, but he did it himself. No one saw. No one knew. What a lesson."

Back in 1974, a few days after I arrived at her home, Mrs. Cohen wanted to welcome me with something special. Probably thinking Japanese love fish, she cooked a large, whole white fish. She beamed, presenting it to the table. The odour and texture repulsed me. I could not eat a nibble and did not know how to tell her.

The work was simple, and they treated me well. At their dinners and parties, I met cultured, important people — politicians, actors, business-people. My boyfriend — an affluent, kind, young American wanted to marry me and take me to the states. This was life in Canada, a nice place, just cold.

In the end, Rusty and I did not share the same values, so we broke up. After a year, I left the wealthy family's home and entered a new reality of daily life.

To survive, I worked three minimum wage part-time jobs. My friends told me: to secure a job in Canada I had to talk myself up. So I marched into Mr. Brooks' dog grooming salon and told him I had experience working with dogs. We always had a dog on the farm and I adore them. That was my experience. Mr. Brooks hired me to bathe the dogs. I found other part-time jobs washing women's hair at a beauty salon and as a chambermaid at a hotel.

I rented a basement room in an old downtown house. An elderly lady shared my fridge, sink, shower, and washroom. My diet was three loaves of raisin bread and a head of cabbage a week. Sometimes I cooked a single pancake in my tiny kitchenette. My grocery budget was twelve dollars a week. Every month I sent money to my sister, Chie, who studied fashion design in Tokyo.

## Measles and kindness, 1975

Every weekend, I drove with other young Calgary Soka Gakkai members over the Rocky Mountains to Seattle for Buddhist youth activities. Depending on road conditions, the drive took thirteen to sixteen hours to reach Seattle. The mountain roads were dangerous and the members' cars in those days were not the safest. So, most weekends we rented cars. Of course, I had to pay my share of the rental, gas, and expenses.

The group prepared for a large conference and festival in Hawai'i that year. They offered me flute lessons since I'd joined their girls' band. In Seattle, we also received spiritual guidance and encouragement in our life struggles. Through these trips, we learned to work together, to challenge and win in our lives.

Our last practice in Seattle was the week before the Hawai'i event. I ran a low fever with a runny nose. The doctor said I had a cold, and I'd be fine for the trip. Usually I got excited hopping in the car with other youthful members, learning about their Canadian life-style and how to swear in English. They coached me on language classes, getting grants to go to school, how to do taxes, and many things. But this time, the trip wasn't so carefree. The fever grew worse. Half-dozing, I slumped in the back seat.

By the time we got to Seattle, I definitely did not suffer from a cold. At once, a local member took me under her broad, powerful wing. Tall with dark chocolate hair in a bun, Bobbie said, "You're coming with me." Through my fever stood a solid tower of women's beauty and power. She poured me into a car and rushed me to the closest hospital.

One glance and the young American doctor said, "*Hashika*," Japanese for measles.

"The rash is starting. You will be very contagious for the next four days. Stay inside and away from children. See your doctor when you get back to Canada."

"I am going to Hawai'i in a week."

"You will still be sick, but not contagious, so long as you depart over four days from today."

Bobbie paid for my medications and the hospital visit without asking. Bobbie and the doctor taught me a lesson in care and consideration. Our paths never crossed again, so I never repaid or thanked her. Since that experience, whenever I have the opportunity, even with strangers, I strive to be kind like Bobbie. That has become my way of thanking her.

A week later, on Waikiki beach, the fever had broken, red blotches blemished my legs. Thousands of members from North America gathered for peace on the island where the Pacific War started. Joining us was a contingent from Hiroshima, where it ended.

## Daddy was dying, Japan

In the winter of 1975–76, my father was dying from pancreatic cancer. By working extra shifts at the hair salon, I'd saved enough for the flight to Tokyo. With holiday hair styling, the salon kept busy, so I collected lots of tips. The owner added her own tips to mine. After the Christmas rush, I flew home to be with Dad for New Year's. With the tip money, I'd buy train tickets from Tokyo to Tottori.

In Tokyo, I stayed the first night at my little sister's place before taking the train home. You hear of these tiny chicken-coop Tokyo apartments? My walk-in closet today is nearly the same size as Chie's entire one-room apartment. No wider than our arms extended. I brought her a suede jacket as a gift. With her skills from school, she'd adjust it to her slight frame.

The next day Chie and I travelled on the bullet train to Okayama, then a local express to Yonago in Tottori Prefecture. On the train, we got caught up. Besides school, she worked part time at a Tokyo bakery.

## Daddy is in hospital, Yonago

Without Chie, I would have gotten lost. Japan seemed foreign, disorienting. Dad stayed in a ward with five other men at the Yonago Tottori University Hospital. Mom slept on the floor beside his bed to take care of him. She brought a futon from home that she rolled up under his bed during the day. Other spouses also stayed in the room. The ward had a common kitchen with three or four coin-operated propane stoves. I'd never noticed this set-up before, or since. Mom slid a ten yen coin in the slot and received a few minutes of propane to cook a meal for her and Dad.

"Yo-chan, you've come? You've come from Canada? You've returned?"

"Daddy, I brought you postcards from Canada. The Rockies. Prairies."

He examined each card. "I won't die in a hospital. After going west, north and south, I'm not gonna die in this hospital."

"We'll bring you home for New Year's. Do you need anything, Daddy? Are you hungry?" He's going to ask for some of that hard, black, Russian bread he loved so much.

"Bamboo shoots. I want to taste bamboo shoots."

Late December was still too early for bamboo to have their babies. If I searched in Yonago, I'd lose my way. Chie and Mom said they'd go. Whatever he wanted, Mom would find and cook. Meanwhile, I stayed with Dad.

After my less than two years in Canada, Japan was a culture shock. Plus, I was jet lagged. I'd already forgotten the little things. When I requested from the ward's nurse if Dad might come home, my body forgot when to bow. My mouth forgot the small polite words it was supposed to say.

I felt ten-years-old. Daddy's horse escaped. With muddy knees and face, I scurried over the fields to fetch dear Dannoko. Ten-years-old, running an errand for Dad, I will bring his horse home. I can do this. I will bring you home, Daddy.

The nurse, starched in lily-white, said, "Of course. He must go home for New Year's."

She led me to the doctor's office. "Honourable Doctor," her body was straight, at attention, "may I present Mr. Yamamoto's daughter from Canada? She wishes to release her father for the New Year's holidays."

"Canada?" He peered at me over his glasses, shuffled papers, and glanced back at the nurse. "Well, it's New Year's. Provide the arrangements for a temporary release."

That was that. She dismissed me. They would contact my brother with details.

I headed back to Dad's room. Mom and Chie hadn't returned. "Daddy, we will take you home before New Year's. I will bake you banana bread in Aino, as we make it in Canada. You will love it." I tidied the room around his bed. He still held the postcards.

"Is Canada really like this?" He turned to his neighbour, awake in the next bed. "My daughter came from Canada to see me. It's so open. I want to go to Canada."

The neighbour looked impressed. The woman with him said, "You've travelled so far."

"Hello," was all I managed.

I assisted him in changing his gown. My hand skimmed over something on his side. A bump? A scar? "Daddy?"

"The Russian guns were much stronger than ours. Our bolt-action Arisakas were no match against the Russian Mosin rifles. You had to stay low. The guy next to me raised his head. A single shot blew off his face. His face exploded over me. I lunged to help him. That's when I spotted my ripped shirt. The bullet grazed me."

"I never knew. How could I not know?"

"Yo-chan, you came home to see me. I might die soon. But we will meet again."

Mom and Chie came back. "Impossible to find fresh bamboo shoots at the end of December. We found pickled."

I caught Dad's eyes and nodded, anticipating what he would say: "Pickled bamboo shoots . . . I remember . . . so tasty with *saké* . . ."

## The broken guitar string, Calgary, 1978

A couple of years later, I had a dream. Sobbing, I woke up, punching Keith. My fists pounded him. "You have a father. What's wrong with you? Your father is alive. *Oto-chan* is gone."

Keith woke, grabbed my hands, held them, held me. "I am so sorry. What happened?"

"I don't know. A dream."

"What do you remember?"

"Nothing. Only a guitar, a six string guitar. One string broke, hanging loose."

"Six? Let's see. You, your mother and father, Chie, and Yusaku. That's five. And another — your oldest brother, who died?"

# after-death in three verses

what are you doing today?
maybe send flowers
We've silence round the kitchen table
and coffee's getting cold.
Memories are slippery

what are you doing today?
the lilacs are blooming
We're gathering round the kitchen table
and coffee cups are raised.
Memories of lost laughter

what are you doing today?
Guess I'll help mow the neighbor's lawn
We're together round the kitchen table
more coffee's being poured,
Memories making us laugh

# "Ask for Yoshiko."

## Leaving Los Angeles, 1976

By 1976, I was a mess. Mom and Dad were also a mess. Dad had taken a position at the University of Calgary. Mom accompanied him back to Canada, but they both had enough. Finally, they split up.

"Come up," he offered on the phone. "Stay with me until you get on your feet. I need the company. Your mother's already gone back to Vancouver."

---

Once again, I met Larry at his Santa Monica office. I told him about casing expensive houses, looking for ways to break in and steal. The way everything had gone wrong, the full confession. He smiled and said, "Yeah, LA can be too much. It's no shame. You will do well in Canada. You are from there, right? I hear Calgary is spectacular, the outdoors, mountains. My wife travelled to Calgary for her work. They have real cowboys, not our movie cowboys. And horses. She says horses held the right-of-way on the city streets." He dug through a directory and found a phone number for a member in Calgary.

Outdoors, cowboys, animals. Not remotely my style. I might be too hasty. Well, it's only for six months or so. Work up north, make money, pull my Buddhist practice back together.

I left Los Angeles with a single suitcase, a box of papers, my Canadian birth certificate and US Passport.

## Cold, free air

As I exited the Calgary airport terminal, the brisk March air wrapped my face, awakening my senses. I drew a deep breath, the deepest in a long time. Biting and fresh, the northern wind blew away the choking, oppressive, smog of LA.

Dad guided me around the city for a couple of days, getting me oriented. The seasons changed and Calgary, the centre of Canada's oil industry, boomed economically. Steel and glass skyscrapers rose under construction everywhere. Streets detoured, high-rise cranes dotted the sky. Snowbanks and dirty slush lined some streets. Grass and trees turned pale-green on others. Didn't spot any cowboys or horses. Calgary resembled a small city being pulled out of a big crate.

Dad pulled the family out of Vancouver's paradise, and further south, always for the sake of his career. Now, he was returning me home, a home I didn't know.

## Lake Louise, 1976

My second day in Calgary, Dad took me into the Rocky Mountains, loaning me his old US Navy deck jacket against the mountain's chill. As we drove higher along the Bow River, lodgepole pine and fir gave way to spruce. The deeper into the mountains and higher he drove, the further back in history we seemed to go.

We followed the CP Rail line into Banff. "The first Chinese built the railway," Dad elaborated. We stood at the head of the Spiral Tunnels, deep railway tunnels circling inside the mountains and across rivers. "On the walls and ceilings, they wrote the Chinese characters for their countrymen who died during construction." The east-west railway proved pivotal to the country's beginnings and survival as a nation. The railway workers' nineteenth century discovery of thermal springs at Banff started the boom of world tourism.

Lake Louise itself was still frozen from winter and blanketed in snow. A grand chateau, from 1890, stood at the lakeside. Glaciers hung above us, millions of years older. They yield current revelations in geology and paleontology and climate. Dad proved a competent tour guide, informative and considerate. This was satisfying. I never heard my father teach, never attended his class. Dad's sole exceptional ability, I missed.

The gentle spring light softened the shadows of the mountains and trees. Skaters glided over the frozen lake; the grinding of their blades scraping ice startled me. Icy air carried the heady scent of spruce trees.

Dad's olive-drab khaki jacket wrapped me in decades of musk and pipe tobacco. More history hid in the coat — salt air, the cordite smell of spent ordnance and half-burned kamikaze gasoline. Wearing his alpaca lined jacket, breathing the mountain air, connected me to Dad at his best.

Dad wore the deck jacket while commanding PCE-848, an escort and mobile hospital ship, from the end of 1944 until decommissioned after the war. After the Japanese surrendered in August 1945, he became "part of a one-day tour by Naval personnel of Hiroshima," he recalled in his memoirs. "I'll never forget the awful smell in the city and the total silence. It was amazing to see the utter and indiscriminate devastation in every direction, and to realize that one bomb had created such incredible destruction. This experience, it turned out, had a huge impact on me. Irrespective of the right or wrong of Japanese behaviour in the war, I was determined to work hard, as a civilian, to do what I could to ensure that such a catastrophe would never happen again."[46]

Dad and Mom came from the greatest generation: regular men and women of every country who dealt a single defeat to fascism. During the war, Dad explained, he became part of something greater than himself. This sense of connection to the events of the day — war, injustice, poverty — remained with Mom and Dad throughout their lives. They always saw themselves as part of their times.

After WWII, they took part in peace campaigns from the late 1940s and in many social justice causes. They grew active in the US civil rights movement. They tried to imbue in me the values of Martin Luther King Jr., quoting: "Life's most persistent and urgent question is: 'What are you doing for others?'"[47]

After everything we'd been through, both our individual troubles and in our conflicts with each other, Dad and I stood on this mountain hanging out. Nice. Two lives in transition. For one afternoon, at least, we faced the unknown together.

## A long dialogue begins, Spring

Those first few days in Calgary, we talked. Sitting in his house, two glasses of The Famous Grouse scotch, John Coltrane on the stereo. Boxes piled here and there: they hadn't finished moving in when Mom left. He had an offer on the place and he started packing out. During the couple of months we shared, Dad and I began an adult dialogue that continued the next forty years. Both of us faced uncertain futures. But for the moment, two broken guys found comfort in each other's presence.

"I've clipped some articles on regional enteritis. Have a look."

"Thanks. It's called Crohn's now, Dad."

"How is your teacher, Ikeda? Still travelling? Still talking with the right people?"

"He's been to China and the Soviet Union, coaxing them to dialogue, not start a war. Last year, he set up a worldwide group at a conference in Guam. We are now part of Soka Gakkai International."

"Guam? Interesting choice. He's doing the right things. What about your priests? Do you still keep temples?" That's nice. Dad cares, showing curiosity.

"Yeah, Dad, we still have priests."

"What do they do? Robes and bells, all that." His legs spread, a slight smile. A sip of scotch.

I twisted on the sofa away from him, defensive, not sure why. "Ceremonies and funerals and, you know, priest stuff."

"They don't chant for you. You do that yourselves?"

"True. Got me there, Pops."

He turned the glass in his hands, leaning towards me, clearing his throat. More than conversation or idle curiosity.

"Keep an eye on them, Keith. How do they really regard Ikeda, his politics, the peace work? Parasites, they will bleed your organisation dry."

What's his interest? Why push this? Probably he'd been doing his academic research, Dad's way of caring for me. "All right, I will. Sounds like you're still keeping an eye on us."

He appreciated that. The smile reappeared, supported by Coltrane's "Favorite Things."

From those days surrounded by moving boxes until I held his hand for one final exhale, we talked and argued and tried to answer pertinent questions. For nearly forty years, I never heard him speak one harsh word about Mom.

## A warm welcome

Lots to do: find a job, a car, a place to live. Start getting my life and practice back together. First things first. I called the number Larry gave me. The lady sounded pleasant, even warm. I introduced myself and told her I was staying at my father's place in Elbow Park. I hoped to become involved, contribute to activities with the local Buddhist organisation. She told me about their small group and gave me details for their gatherings.

I said, "Since I'm here, I'll need to get a job."

Pause. "Of course."

Then something else. "Since I need to get a job, I have to get my hair cut."

Her warm voice turned wary. "Yes?"

"Just wondering if you know anywhere near here that gives good haircuts."

"Actually, I do. Go to the Magic Beauty Salon. It's on Fifteenth Avenue and Fourth Street, not far from you. Ask for Yoshiko."

## Magic Beauty Salon

Two days later, wearing Dad's Navy coat in the spring chill, I walked to the hair salon. An Asian lady greeted me at the entrance.

Yoshiko is a Japanese name. This lady is Asian; she must be Yoshiko. Clever me.

"I'm looking for Yoshiko."

"Yoshiko isn't here."

"Oh, when does she work?"

"Not until Saturday."

"Okay, can I book with her for Saturday?"

"No, she doesn't cut hair."

Still standing at the entrance, I peered inside. This is a hair salon. Row of chairs under those stainless steel can-things that go over women's heads. The alcohol odour of hair spray and antiseptic. Weird. I am requesting a haircut from a person who doesn't cut hair. For an instant, I imagined the rack of women's magazines hid a secret door. This place is a front for a super secret spy ring. "Ask for Yoshiko" might be code and I am hunting for a dangerous (and beautiful) international assassin. For an instant.

"She is the shampoo girl. She works once a week. You can't make an appointment with her."

"Oh. Okay." Too embarrassed now to request a haircut and oddly disappointed, I forced a smile. It made sense, sort of. But weird. A few days ago, at home in LA, and now standing at the entrance of a beauty salon in Canada, asking for someone named Yoshiko.

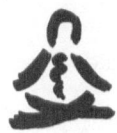

# I Will Never Forget His Eyes.

## An unusual young man

ONE EVENING IN MARCH 1976, a newcomer came to our Buddhist meeting. Around ten people gathered for a regular gathering in the living room of a member's apartment. First, we recited our evening prayers. The newcomer didn't hesitate; he recited the sutra along with us, so he must be a member. After chanting came the discussion period. The way he walked, I'd never met such a person. More than a strut, this guy stomped. Parading from the back of the room to speak at the front, a man racing towards a goal. His bell bottoms had stitches down the seams and his legs jumped at every step. Over his shoulder hung a purse. It swung as he swayed his arms. What man has a purse? He introduced himself to everybody; actually he announced his arrival. Even as he stood and spoke, declaring he'd come from LA, his arms swung and legs stepped in place. Clearly, he wanted attention. The word pompous wasn't in my vocabulary yet.

## A proposal, February 1977

A year later, he invited me for dinner. Our first date. At the restaurant, he proposed. "The reason I invited you out is I want to marry you. If you say yes, I'll be happy. If you say no, I understand. Please say yes." What a proposal. What an attitude. What a first date. He impressed me by knowing what he wanted, and he pursued it.

I had so many questions, most for myself. My brain rolled round and round as I sat at the restaurant table. I didn't answer him. In fact, I said nothing. I sat silent.

So, he asked me again to marry him. Except this time, louder.

Loud enough for the other diners to hear. I felt so embarrassed. I stayed silent.

And he repeated himself. This time slower.

I said, "I need time. I need to chant about this."

He said he understood. We finished dinner. I had to pay my half. He drove me home. In the car, my mind still going round and round. He'd stunned me. At the same time, Keith had something that attracted me. He was committed to our faith. I wanted to talk with Mom. I needed to get home to chant.

As we got closer to my apartment, I recognized his nervousness. He dropped me off. He wasn't going to try for a kiss.

Actually, Keith wasn't the first to propose. Several boys wanted to marry me. This one came across differently, though. Deep inside, I trusted my faith and, although I didn't understand him, sensed we shared the same direction in life.

I chanted and chanted, then phoned Mom. In those days, a phone call to Japan meant a huge deal. I waited until Sunday evening after five when overseas calls were half off. On reflection, it's good I didn't tell her every detail. I didn't tell her I had to pay for half the dinner. "Mom, there is a guy from America. Comes from a Jewish family. His father is a professor here. He has faith and is committed to our practice." I gave her the impression Keith was a together young man.

Mom told me of her nightmare: I stood abandoned at a dirty crossroad with a child in hand, piles of suitcases and nowhere to go, with her too far away to aid. Mom thought of Manchuria. Nobody had aided her, not her husband, not her mother. "I am far away and can't come to assist you. Flying overseas would be all but impossible. I trust your decision. You can take care of yourself, your life with this person." And again, "I trust you, Yo-chan."

I phoned an older married friend, who knew us both, requesting her advice. She had warned me off the others, counselling, "If you are going to be with somebody, make sure you share common values." But this time she said, "Keith is a good person."

Certainly, I needed to understand him better. Maybe this was a guy who could be my comrade, support me to achieve my goals in Canada. I had many doubts about him, but found myself connected to him.

## Meeting Ira and Irene

Soon after that, we visited Keith's father at his new girlfriend's house. We sipped coffee and she baked me a cake. Ira acted nice, and I accepted his queries. "Why are you interested in my son?"

"I trust his faith."

A few days later, Keith said he was proud of me for saying that. "My Dad phoned, asking over and over what that means, you trust my faith."

Ira invited us to an elegant event, a fancy art opening. It turned out a double-date. We dressed up for a night on the town. I enjoyed the evening. Hors d'oeuvres and corsages. Again, under inspection. Ira scrutinized my behaviour at this lavish event. He treated me like a student, an unusual student. He tested me, but that was him. Keith and I enjoyed a great time.

## Can he make you happy? Vancouver

We flew to Vancouver to meet Keith's mother. She was getting settled after her divorce, renting an old house. Irene organized the small house and set up a room for us. On shelves were knick-knacks, a few from Asia. She spoke of her love for Asia and her Japanese friends, like a collector describing their treasures. My plans didn't include becoming a cute Japanese doll for display on her shelf.

She made a couple of dips for snacks — eggplant baba ganoush and guacamole. Pretty hip for those days. Keith busied himself reading her *New Yorker* magazines. Once she had me alone, she showed me the backyard and talked of the garden she planned to grow. We shared a love of plants and gardening. I envied all she'd grow in Vancouver's friendly climate. Her questions turned personal. "Can he make you happy?" "Does he make you happy in bed?" I figured she tried to shock me or impress me. "You know Keith is not well; you can't count on him."

I didn't know. Keith told me about a disease. I didn't understand the details, but it sounded as though all was well. At the time, his health seemed fine, other than the long leaking scar on his belly.

She drove us to Granville Island Market, where she insisted we buy a beautiful fresh piece of tuna. "You can prepare sushi." She couldn't know; she didn't ask — in those days, I detested fish and meat. We returned to the house with the tuna and I tried to remember how Mom prepared fish.

She enjoyed living in Vancouver, but she also needed to figure out what to do with her life. Everybody's life was shifting.

Meeting the parents is a serious event in Japan, as in Canada, indicating commitment, filled with the stress of first impressions. None of the other boys who proposed took me to meet their families. Visiting Keith's mother and father, I didn't feel like the outsider going to meet the family alone. Keith and I were together visiting them. He stood on my side, making me comfortable. We were side by side. I liked that. I enjoyed sharing a sense of purpose with Keith. We had fun on our first steps together.

## Would we make it? 1977–1980

Keith and I were learning about each other. He was so focussed and determined. One evening, he came over to my apartment. By then I shared a proper apartment with a friend, not the basement with the elderly lady. He cooked steak and broccoli with a fancy sauce for me and my roommate. They enjoyed the steaks. I ate the veggies, scraping off the sauce. He told my roommate he'd be moving in and could she please leave? Really. He announced his intention to help her pack and move.

We didn't understand each other, but a future with him excited me. He spoke nicely. My English wasn't good. He would take care of me. He said he would.

Just before our wedding, he lost his job. He got another job. It didn't last. The path ahead looked rocky. Keith lost or quit jobs. Keith also was naïve. Intelligent and good-hearted, but he needed to learn adult responsibility.

He loved Ikeda-sensei and our Buddhist movement. We'd advance together. Through our faith and practice, we'd create a beautiful life, build a harmonious family, and show others a way to peace.

Losing jobs shocked him, but not enough. He still didn't see. What did he think? The world owed him a living? Even though we were poor, he gave money away to charities, paying a friend's rent, or a beggar on the street. If anyone needed a place to stay, he volunteered our couch.

But I questioned, were we able to make it? Why carry on with this guy for a lifetime? I might be better off on my own.

We had other issues too, like any new couple. I said nothing. He should understand me, my heart. It took me too long to figure out — I had to speak up for myself, for our new family's sake.

## Teeth

With no training, credentials, or experience, I fell into my profession. Around 1976, I quit my part-time job at the hotel and got another part-time job at a small accounting firm. I never studied accounting, and I still didn't speak English well enough to take care of customers. So, I only did odd jobs around the office — dusting, preparing coffee, filing. The owner, Ben, appreciated the way I worked, but after a few months, said: "Yoshiko, I don't have enough for you to do. You focus and are good with your hands. Ever thought of working in a dental lab? One of our clients is a small lab and they often need technicians." Ben drove me to this laboratory near my place.

Ben left me at the lab and they let me spend the day watching the technicians work. The dental lab looked like nothing I'd seen. Individual powerful furnaces, electric grinders, and polishing devices surrounded each technician's station. Rows of tubes filled with porcelain powder in dozens of shades sat on shelves next to bottles of precious and semi-precious metals. All day, I observed, amazed and fascinated.

The technicians resembled artists and factory workers, and craftspeople, all in one. They were like potters; instead of bowls, they built teeth out of porcelain and metal. The colours had to be perfect, the shape, precise.

What to ask, other than, "what are you doing?" Or, "what is that tool?" Several of the technicians bragged about their certificates and years of training. They were contrary, dismissive of me. Who is this immigrant girl who can't even speak English?

After, in the lab owner's office, "So, what do you think?"

"I can try."

The job demanded physical and mental concentration and exposed my eyes and hands to dangerous chemicals. At first, my colleagues criticized me, saying "you don't have a technician's licence or certificate. Your skills will never be good enough. You only got this job because the bosses play favourites." They protected their achievements and grew jealous. Despite their criticisms, I enjoyed the work. To hold a proper job made me so happy instead of bouncing around working part time.

I pursued whatever training became available and consistently received large pay increases. Later, with Keith losing jobs and the girls arriving, we survived only because of my job. The job became my pride and our sole stable point in the approaching challenges. Nothing stopped me; I became a moving train. I stuck to it for over thirty years.

## Meeting our mentor, 1981

Together with Keith and twenty two-month-old Erica, I flew to Toronto. Keith's health, our finances, our relationship remained shaky. We seemed to be on the edge of collapse. We wished to help welcome Mr. and Mrs. Ikeda on their visit to Canada. Keith volunteered behind the scenes; he did not attend the big general meeting.

In Toronto, Erica ran around the Harbour Castle Conference Centre, out of control. Of course, the long plane ride exhausted her. She grew cranky by the minute. Other children ran around as well, yelling and being kids. I'd flown to Toronto to help. Instead, we threatened to disturb the event. The trip looked like it would be a waste of time.

Someone ushered us mothers and children to a back room, behind the main hall, where we would not interrupt the activity.

After the meeting, sensei came to the room where we waited. For an instant, he caught my eye; he placed his hand on Erica's and other children's heads and chanted three times for each child. I will never forget that moment. Time stood still. A calm orbit of care and compassion wrapped my stress and troubles.

I'd met famous people, politicians, athletes, celebrities. Some were warm, but I'd never had that feeling of being seen, of being understood, and trusted. The moment of compassion for me and Erica taught me a lesson: everybody, everywhere, Canada, and the world needs compassion. Erica and I must grow to contribute to others' happiness. We had to win.

When later I found out sensei had been ill in Toronto, I was overcome with emotion. Even when sick, we can live with kindness and help others.

## A dance of faith

Between Erica and Andrea, I miscarried. I was around two and a half months pregnant. Keith had gone out of town, encouraging members in Saskatchewan. I drove Erica, then two, to the car wash. I hefted the heavy overhead door to the car wash, feeling its weight. Maybe washing the car wasn't a good idea. Late that night, Keith came home. The pain started. Then bleeding. We rushed to emergency.

They told me the baby had already passed. They admitted me and performed a dilation and curettage. The doctor said normally they advise waiting six months to become pregnant again. In my case, we could try again once I had a regular cycle. Even though they said nothing was wrong with me, a thousand times my mind replays lifting that heavy door.

The pain of losing my child never fades away. It is a pain that unites me with every parent who has lost a child. My eldest brother starved to death before age one. The Kato's babies. All the lost children: red dragonflies, now dead, only memories in song.

Andrea came quickly, around ten months later. We took part in Soka Gakkai activities most every night with the girls. We bought an old, falling apart inner city house — less than 600 square feet for us four and a cat. To fit attendants for Buddhist gatherings, we carried the furniture out onto the front lawn. Members and guests sat on the faded sixties green carpet.

Keith and I were in a dance of faith and purpose. We stumbled a lot and stepped on each other's toes. Others criticised us: We'd never own a nice place to live. Keith is a bum. You will carry him forever. Can't he buy you nice clothes?

I thought, I will show the critics. I will win. Whatever it takes, I will fulfill my vow, create a happy, harmonious family, and contribute to Canadian society.

When we were not having gatherings in our home, we travelled around Canada and the western US for activities. The girls went with us everywhere. In the car for twelve or fourteen hours, we listened to my blues tapes and Keith's jazz.

Every time we made a fresh start, Keith lost his job or had to be hospitalized. Over and over. As if I had every trouble possible. In my letters home to Mom, I left out some surgeries. I hated to make her more worried.

## Becoming who I am, 1987

Eventually, we bought a larger house to hold larger meetings. Our house became the centre for our Buddhist activities for the province until the group built a proper centre. We welcomed so many into our home. Wonderful, fascinating people; and a few who were not so wonderful.

I learned from everybody — wealthy and poor, arrogant priests, many artists, and regular folk. Their behaviour taught more than their words. Each has assisted me in becoming who I am today.

The girls joined our dance of faith and purpose and supported our advance. They taught us to parent, to listen to others. All the normal experiences of every Canadian parent became, for Keith and me, opportunities to learn. I grew up in a different culture. Keith grew up so isolated, in many ways in a different world. We had wisdom from our practice but lacked common sense, basic living savvy. Parent-teacher interviews, birthday parties, skating and dance classes are normal family experiences. For Keith and me, they were lessons. The girls had childhoods and relationships, foreign to us. The girls taught us who we are, through their mirroring. We paid attention to their voices, their behaviour, their eyes. Their relationship with each other differed from mine with Chie and Yusaku. Erica and Andrea taught me about myself and assisted me in empathising with others.

The girls worked through the usual pre-teen and teen experiences. Boyfriend troubles. Their friends' boyfriend troubles. And school troubles and troubles at home. Normal, but for Keith and I, foreign. Our teen years were so different; we needed to learn through theirs.

Lots of unexpressed assumptions remained between us. We're still learning to communicate clearly with each other instead of assuming. We are still dancing and still stepping on each other toes.

Financially, our situation has completely improved. Now, Keith is still as generous towards others, even more so, but not as impulsive. He is the most responsible person, tracking every penny, frugal with our money. We plan our retirements together, decide together.

We live in an attractive, spacious house now. Visitors say, "Your house is so beautiful."

Keith's response is always the same: "The world has lots of beautiful houses. What is important is the actions inside the house. Is there laughter and joy? Are the inhabitants kind, caring, and generous?"

Others who witnessed our experience expressed appreciation for all our struggles. We gave them hope, modelling latitude, commitment, and determination.

# The Striving

## The milkmaid, Kingdom of Magadha, 445 BCE

A MILKMAID FOUND SIDDHARTHA collapsed on the banks above the Nairañjanā river. Physically and mentally spent, options exhausted, the man who sought freedom had run out of choices. She offered him rice gruel, the soft taste of yoghurty porridge, and the touch of a human hand. He ate, drank, then bathed in the river. Her name was Sujata. We learn his teachings today because of her, her dog, her porridge.

## Sujata's story

Of course, I remember the man. The pariah dog found him, not me. Its barking saved him, really. That spring morning began beautifully, just before the full moon. The pastures grew pea green fresh. I'd finished milking the girls and packed up to take them to pasture. The pariah led the bulls to water up the Nair'. That's the way it goes, you see. The bulls pasture while the cows milk. You must keep them separate, especially in the spring, or you'll get nothing but trouble. It's not hard once you know how, and you're blessed with a strong back, and you get help with the herding from the pariah.

I cooked *payasa* porridge for my morning meal. To celebrate the day before the blossom moon, I even mixed cooked rice in with the curds and a leaf of cardamom. I'd enjoy a spring feast sitting under the giant, gnarled banyan tree while the herd grazed. Boss lady says I should pray to the spirit in that old tree for a husband, but I'm not sure.

Anyway, I never got to the banyan that day, not for feasting, nor praying, nor just for shade. The barking of the pariah would have raised the dead.

He was howling, I'm telling you, wild as a cyclone. I bolted towards the river, figuring an ox got itself hurt.

In the quag above the banks, I found the animal licking and barking and nudging the body of a man. He lay half sunk in mud, unshaven, hair long and dirty and untied. The man's robe, tattered and soiled, had a patch or two of dirty yellow. Yellow. One of those wise wanderers. A fool wanderer, more likely. Starved himself. More than likely thinking if light enough, he'd float to heaven. That's the way those fools think. So busy destroying their own body, they lose their minds as well.

Oh, he was in rough, rough shape, ribs sticking out like the rafters of a broken barn. His hair, like brittle straw, fell out to my touch. My hand gripped right round his leg. To think he did this to himself. To think he thought it right to do this to himself. But he wasn't dead, not yet. The dog licked his fingers, and they twitched. He faded fast, on the very edge. Like I say, the dog was trying to raise the dead.

And he weighed near nothing. Don't mistake me for some precious princess in a song. Me and the pariah dog carried and dragged him to the Nairañjanā.

Got water into him and he came around, bit by bit. Muttering wild talk in an odd accent. A demon, or a voice from the other side, spoke through him. He mumbled about an apple tree, liberation, suffering. He may have uttered "*Ammā*, mama." Who knows? Spirit's talk.

"No fruit trees this side of the Nair', Sir," I told him. "Pipals on the far side, but no apples this far south, as best I know." That accounted for the accent, speaking of apple trees. He must be from up north, travelled here to die in mud and reeds and cow dung.

"Pipal trees?" He demanded, "Show me."

"No, Sir. You step in the river, the way you are, you'll wash away like a leaf. First, get some food into you. I made rice *payasa* from my girls' spring milk. Hey, come back. Wake up now."

We were losing the man. The pariah whimpered, turning in circles, tail tucked. I made out some words, "All has failed... find a way out of misery and discontent... for everyone..." The man fought hard, don't get me wrong, but something mean pulled him beyond.

The poor dog was shaking, howling now, as if the animal's own gods whelped through him. The lady says don't talk cross to menfolk, respect your betters, but pity said it; I did. What else could I do? "You holy men think it is a sin to feed the body? You need the body, same as the spirit, no less. By the gods, let's sit you up. Please, sir, open your mouth. Please, you must eat. You want to save all, let me save you."

My fingers shook. I remember. He'd stopped mumbling, stopped breathing. Pulling him up to my lap. The terns were shrieking, the herons booming. The sun blazed off the river, stinging my eyes. No boats on the Nair'. Nobody around. Just me and the pariah yowling and this man's empty body cradled in my arms. My clothes and his rags tangled. My hair fell into his, braiding with his sickly locks like the edging of a rug; sweat and sand blinded my eyes. Both of us now wrapped in dung and sweat and mud. Holding him up. Forcing open his fool mouth. Drawing the porridge out of my kit without spilling, blind. My fingers in his mouth. Yeah, I remember.

---

His mumbling returned. "Where are the ascetics?"

"You dreaming again, Sir?"

"My companions."

It seemed a holy vision struck him, still talking mad. The man's alone. But the dog started growling, so I scanned round and spotted them hiding and spying from behind the tall grass. Five of them. Skeletons, wearing barely a stitch for modesty. Not raising a single bony finger to rescue this poor man. These are his friends?

## The five ascetics

The five ascetics were disgusted, observing him eat, watching him break his vows of self-denial. "This imposter has grown decadent in his ways and given up the struggle. We will never listen to him." They abandoned him, leaving only the echoes of their curses.

Sujata found an inlet of the river where the current slowed so he could bathe safely. He'd lost his knife, so she loaned him her iron blade while she headed back to her herd and chores. She also left him the jar with the remains of the porridge. Hours later, she returned to find the empty jar and her blade atop a pile of hair and beard.

## Against the flow

A wee something in his belly revitalized him and the bath cleared his mind. The bath seemed to rinse away the ascetic practices, the chatter of competing dogmas. Refreshed, alone again, and possibly wiser, he continued south along the left bank, arriving at a ford across from a grove.

The grove sat outside a village called Uruvelā along the Nairañjanā River in the kingdom of Magadha. (Today, the name of the village is Bodh Gaya, village of enlightenment, in the Indian state of Bihar.)

Peering across the river, he spotted a majestic fig tree in the centre of the grove. The pipal's branches spread in welcome. Skimmers and terns squeaked and chirped. The birds' calls reminded him of the music of the minstrels, the sound of life and creation. Their flapping wings carried the vibration to his ears and beyond. Now, to cross the river. The pipal offered a seat for his last battle, triumphant or defeated.

He stepped off the bank. The riverbed was soft mud. The river at first only reached his calves, but the current was swift. He swayed and steadied himself. As Sujata predicted, the current threatened to sweep him away with the leaves.

Nay, I am not a leaf. I am a person, an ordinary person. And like all people, I possess will, intention, and determination. If I so choose, I go against the current. I will achieve what none before have. Or drown.

He imagined a leaf floating on the river, floating away from him, gracefully upstream, against the flow. That is how I will be. I will cross with ease.

All meditations and disciplines had been in vain — dead ends. He struggled ahead against the current. Vanity, now gone, floated away downstream. Siddhartha stumbled a few steps forward in the river. Once again, alone with his angst — how to live fully in a world where the only certainty is death. He sensed a resolve in his chest and in the pit of his stomach. Follow the milkmaid — choose kindness, lucidity, and purpose instead of hatred, greed, delusion. Find a compassionate way to be in this fluid suffering existence or perish trying. Let only bones remain, he would not cease his quest.

Determined or no, a person's legs must move. Imaginings of ease or no, an ordinary person must step. During the winter the Nairañjanā's flow declined; its bank widened. Now, the spring snow melt off the Himalayas pushed the current, low and fast. The waxing moon urged the waters faster. The soft muddy riverbed shifted and sunk underfoot. One moment the mud clung to his feet, like death's wet lips sucking him to doom. The next, the river bottom slipped, making traction and footing impossible. The racing now thigh-high current threatened to topple him. He'd picked the only possible spot to cross — a ford named Suppatittha. In fact, he was crossing during the year's first flood. No god, miracle, or ferry will carry me. I am no god, command no miracles. I must be the ferry.

Step by buffeted, slippery step, Siddhartha crossed the Nairañjanā. He crumbled to his knees on the far side. A local farmer met him crawling on all fours over a sandbank. I don't know the farmer or his wife's name; their deeds deserve telling.

## The farmer's story

Sure we spot wandering hobos, since we are on the river about two *yojanas* north of the Great Trunk Road. Occasionally, a lost peddler strays off the road to Dobhi.

This fellow was different. His accent, for one. Rarely hear the Kosalan round these parts. Not just the accent; he spoke feverishly, words of battle and salvation. Starved, sickly, barely made it across the Nair'. But only so much I can do. The country is full of the hungry and the sick. His eyes, though. They burned maroon and hazel... fierce.

Mumbled about heading for the pipals. That made sense; rest under the trees. But no, he proclaimed he'd sit until he "found relief from suffering," "triumph or perish." He sounded serious, not crazy. Maybe both.

I offered him a mat the missus wove of munja grass to sit on. Little did I know the battle he'd take on. The World-Honoured One, they call him now. But that afternoon, just before the blossoming full moon, I had no idea. What do I know? The missus and I grow some vegetables, raise a few hens, goats, cows.

## Under the tree

Siddhartha advanced to the pipal tree and, with his back to its generous trunk, faced east. Taking his seat on the farmer's mat, he determined not to rise until he had realised his goal. He must either find purpose in this existence, with all its trauma, or perish. He'd left family and country for this moment. Victory or death. His whole body quivered as he lowered himself, as if Mother Earth herself trembled.

---

He sat. The remains of his patched robe, dirty ochre, stained green and brown by years of mud and grass, mirrored the cow paddocks, fields, and river beyond. As his meditation started, he did not struggle, he sat simply, torso straight, thighs grounded. After all the stresses and abuse, his mind concentrated, now curious, resolute. Under the majestic tree, he heard the water of the Nairañjanā as it flowed.

He sat, attentive and determined. His legs crossed, soles upward on opposite thighs, hands resting on his lap, left hand over right, palms upward and thumbs touching. A human body dwelt in the spring.

He did not use visualisations nor any of the breath techniques he'd learned. The here and now became the object of his focus. His legs and hips rooted to the supportive Earth. From hips, his torso extended erect, limber, and open. He did not take stock, or judge. Nor did he wait for revelation. He attended the moment.

Here was the outline of his body in space, his thinned trunk reaching up and out of his waist, his legs touching the mat. He heard his breath, even and slow, without striving to control it. His heart rhythmically beat in his chest, his entrails processing the remains of Sujata's meal. And deeper, he became aware of his blood flowing in through veins to his heart, out in arteries to the kidneys, and fluid from the kidneys into his bladder. He was conscious of his hands on his lap, skin against the tattered rags and against the cool spring air.

The sounds of the Nairañjanā River flowing and lapping against its banks wafted to his ears. A colony of migratory skimmers and terns bred in the open sand bank on the tree's side of the river. A breeze rustled through the grasses and the tree's leaves. In the branches, a male monkey peered down at the curious sight of the motionless man. A pair of orange billed geese paused in their rounds to regard him seated with eyes closed.

He paid attention to his primordial unease. He listened, finally and fully, to the tooth that ached since childhood. Denial of self led to a dead end. Succumbing to pleasure led to a dead end. Even practising monasticism and self-righteous piety came to nought, another prideful vanity.

The unawakened cling to a fixed self: a warrior, a lover, a king, a wise man. The five ascetics denied the self. A third path appeared before his closed eyes. He accepted his dynamic, contingent self, neither defending its ego nor attacking its existence. Of course we harbour a self. It just isn't what we think it is. Transient, interdependent, becoming.

The afternoon sun heated the spring air against his skin. As dusk fell, the sun setting, the full moon not yet risen, he sensed a resistance, a presence. He was not alone. Something stirred, or he stirred it awake, something old and dark and menacing and familiar. The Devil King Mara, the killer, materialized under the tree, standing before him. Mara, an immortal deity, towered over the seated, destitute man.

## Mara's story

I was minding my business, looking after things, when I spotted this pathetic guy under the tree. Look, I'll be honest, I'd had an eye on him for what, six years or so. Watched him moping around, getting into his arguments, his debates, going round in circles. But now, under the tree, he was in a bind. It made sense to reach out, offer aid for his troubles. Maybe send him back to his pretty little wife and kid, if they'd take him.

He had some wild ideas of "supreme enlightenment," "liberation." Sure. He dreams of saving the world? He's not going to save anyone, starving under a tree. Let's be honest, he was a mess. I just wanted to help.

So, I said to him, "You really looking to do some good? Relax a little. You need to rest. Lemme take care of you." That's what I do: take care of people, watch over things. Let people believe they are in control. They need that feeling. I know better. They need keepers to care for them. Keep things from falling out of line. And this punk was getting close to the line. That won't do.

I took pity on him; he was darn sick and weak. If that cow-bitch and her cur hadn't meddled, he'd be mine already, shovelling dung in hell.

---

The Devil Mara now sat right next to him. Mara sat cross-legged on a grass mat, confiding in his ear, in his head, inside him. Mara spoke in a kind voice, with words reasonable. "You are almost dead. You are as thin as a skeleton, pale as a ghost. A thousand parts dead. One part alive. Live, brother. Live the holy life and do good. I offer you the one part of a thousand, life forever to reap the benefits of goodness."

The Devil and the Buddha are ever side by side within us. "Buddha" means the inner forces of creation and compassion. "Mara" is the capacity to degrade, narrow, deny our own or other's noble agency.

The struggle for freedom, for civilisation and culture never ends. Mara never sleeps. The Buddha must be ever awakening. Centuries later, Nichiren wrote, "Good and evil have been inherent in life since time without beginning."[48]

Mara's offer was nothing extraordinary. Return to who he was, the heir to the Shakya clan, go back to a normal regime, complete normal tasks, be a man like other men. Say farewell to the relentless angst. Lose the pain in his tooth. Simply go back to sleep.

Siddhartha's mindful observing gave way to a full-fledged battle. Inside Siddhartha, he battled doubt, exhaustion, temptation. His doubts, in the end, were not about birth or death or meaning, but his own worth. Was he a product of culture, family, birth? Was destiny decided by God or karma or chance? Or could he step out of myth and the supernatural and live within history, with all its uncertainty and flux? Who was he?

Surrounded by Mara's armies of fear, doubt, sloth, false fame, craving: "I see you, trickster. Your devices change with the winds. There, you ride at the head of all your sour armies — fear, temptation, petty cravings. I sortie forth to battle you directly, wielding the sword of faith in the dignity of every child of Mother Earth. All your armies will not defeat me.

"Devil King, my brother, you speak words at times reasonable, at times threatening, honeyed, bitter, or sour. In all cases, your purpose is to weaken my resolve, to degrade, and diminish. Know this, Lord Mara, you who impede life's flow: just as the taste of the great ocean is ever salty, so the taste of the great dharma is freedom. Freedom will be mine and all beings'. This is my vow and no god or devil or man will sway me."

Siddhartha detected, faced, and attended the weaknesses within him, each of the so-called armies of Mara. And observed as each dissipated, floating away, empty clouds in the evening sky.

## Eventide

In the darkening sky above his closed eyes, the full moon grew on the unseen horizon, the full moon of spring's second month. High overhead night herons passed, flying to foraging sites in the darkness.

He settled. Not in a trance or altered state, he became more aware and present than ever. He discerned exactly where he was, the contours of his body sitting in space. He heard the insects chirping, the wind and river flowing. A solitary bullfrog by the river called ceaselessly for a mate. Its lonely croaking echoed through the night.

He did not meditate on God or holiness. No, his attention, like a beam through a burning glass, fixed on this human, earthly moment. This moment contains all the pasts that came before. This moment contains body and mind, self and environment, living and dying, heaven and hell.

He sat upright, his back straight, but not stiff. He sat through the night, attending to the moment. This moment holds the inevitability of passing. Each birth, destined to die. Each crest has a trough. Steadily, gradually, he passed even the battle. This moment, too, he found, holds the possibility of creation, holds all possibilities.

Choices opened before his shut eyes. Moment by moment, his body formed and dissolved and re-formed. Breath, pulse, digestion; all fluid, being born, craving, dying. In his mind, thoughts emerged and vanished in succession. His space, the night sky, revolved over the sleeping grove and grasses, the flowing river. All things spun in motion, revealing options upon options, three thousand possibilities opened in each moment.

He continued examining the moment, observing his body, mind, self, his place on the mat, his breath, heartbeat, wind through the grove, night animals scurrying. Three sambar doe deers forded the river, searching for suitable stags. They paused in their nocturnal hunt to examine, sniff, and ponder the man.

He sat resolved, but without expectation. Something shifted again. A gradual sense of safety grew in him. His still weakened body far from recovered, he perched at the precipice of ultimate failure. But, here, now, he was safe. The ground and the air and the tree and the night creatures held him.

Embraced by the earth below, the tree, and space, Siddhartha both remained and became. He remained a child of the Shakyas, the product of his father's seed and mother's egg, the product of history and choices. His doubts about worth, roles, meaning, remained present, as leaves falling from the tree remained present, as footprints in the mud. At the same moment, he became the product of his creation, his intention, wisdom, his vow. Remaining and becoming, he could be thus.

# The Awakening

**Gaya, India**

Endless becoming. Continuous fading away. Blossoming and opening. Decomposing and regenerating. A cosmos unfolding and enfolding. This is the anguish and the beauty of nature, our revolving universe. Siddhartha meditated upon it all, witnessed it, contained it all — the macro and the micro in each breath. Alone he sat under a fig tree, a singular spot on the surface of spinning planet Earth.

He no longer struggled with his angst — to confront, without despairing, the misery of existence. Nor was he able to let go of this existential struggle, no easier than letting go of the curve of his elbow, the beat of his heart.

Without struggling or letting go, what remained? Finally and fully, he welcomed himself, a lone seeker with all his doubts. Allowing life as it is, creation as it is, he made room, under the tree, for suffering. He welcomed himself into his story. In accommodating himself, embracing himself, he found room for others.

Let life in, the suffering and the joy. Listen to it. Embrace it fully.

In that moment, the infinite variety of creation emerged. Like light through a drop of dew, life-in-the-moment sparkled into a rainbow. Around him, with the inevitability of day following night, life-force dawned. Within him, life-force emerged, unfurling from inside Siddhartha. Life-force rises and ever fades, ungraspable and as real as the Nairañjanā flowing past his tree, flowing still.

Life-force arose without and within. Possibility included hope. Land, the air, proceed from causality and possess wisdom, a kind of intelligence. His quest began with the inevitability of misery and discontent. Now, in front of his eyes, existence functioned through kindness, mercy. Compassion became an element of being, as were his lungs breathing, his nails growing. He and the world, as real as real can be.

The blossoming moon crossed the meridian, bathing the sky. Only this moment and forward existed. He must not go back.

He grasped the connectedness of all things, all people. We depend upon each other, we arise out of each other, we give rise to each other. Every action we take has effects wide and long. And thus he finally knew, nothing was wasted; what we do matters. Indeed, he now comprehended, what we do matters dearly. His lips curved upwards: what we do matters.

## A kid is born

The farmer who gave Siddhartha the grass mat made by his wife woke before dawn. He did not disturb her sleeping and headed out in the gleam of the full blossoming moon. They'd had a late night. A nanny came due to deliver, her leaking started, eyes in a birthing trance. They'd gone to bed before she started labour. Today must be busy, may as well catch an early start, make use of the full moon's light.

He first checked the goats' pen. The nanny foaled sometime in the night. The new kid suckled heartily. The farmer decided, full moon or not, we won't be sacrificing an animal today. The gods can find their own meal.

He left the mother and newborn and proceeded to the paddock. The cows had also risen early and grazed freely on the dew streaked grasses. Egrets from the wetlands below joined the cattle, feasting on insects disturbed by the cows' hooves. From a rise in the paddock, he peered into the grove of pipal trees. He made out the silhouette of the strange young man from yesterday, still seated upright, unmoved against the great tree.

The farmer started back to the hut, halting to check the hens. It had been a fortunate night. Neither monkeys nor pythons stole any of their birds. In the pale pre-dawn glow, using a basket kept in the chicken pen, he gathered their eggs, spotted and cocoa and tan.

He brought the eggs to his wife, now awake and building a fire outside in the straw and mud oven for their morning meal. Eggplant, peas, and spinach lay prepared to go into an earthenware pot with rice and water. Hoes, spades, and a scythe leaned against the wall behind her.

"One kid arrived. Looks healthy." He reported. "The nanny could use molasses water."

"Buck or doe?" She asked.

"I didn't check. It was dark."

The farmer paused before returning to his chores. The full moon, the newborn goat, the stranger seated throughout the night under the great fig tree. He decided. "Put on an extra bowl, wife. We've a guest. You eat your share. He can eat half o' mine. A new day is here."

## Mother Earth testifies

But the sun of the new day had still not risen. Mara, the devilish function, still lurked, ever present. Mara, the killer, can not be killed. Digging the deepest doubts:

"Who are you to claim this seat? You are nothing, a self-absorbed, doomed drifter. What entitles you to the supreme enlightenment? It is not for you; you deserve nothing. Nobody will testify for you. Nobody cares about you. You abandoned everybody and everybody has rejected you. You disgust everyone, even that smug bitch who married you. Your own mother could not be with you. You failed. Again."

As if in response, Siddhartha's right hand twitched. Still deep in concentration, he slid it out from under the left, carefully raised it from his lap and out to the side. The fingers pointed down, trembling, stretching down past the woven mat. He felt the russet earth below.

"Trickster Mara, you may masquerade behind a thousand masks, but I penetrate them all. I see through your temptations — the bliss of sleep, the grandiosity of power, the certainty of control. You may flatter, cajole, insult. I know your ruse. I choose now to awaken. Here, Evil One, my twin, here is my witness:

"She is my witness. See brother, our mother is here. Prithvi Mata, Mother Earth, testifies to this awakening. The great earth connects us here under this tree to every tree, all homes, to my home."

Above him, Venus rose in the eastern sky, leading the dawn. He drew an immense inhale, his mouth opened, and out poured a primal roar, the lion's roar. He roared in joyous celebration of the dawn: "It is done. I am awake. Dawn breaks as I awaken. My mind is at peace!"

## The first morning

In that moment, alone, near-naked, emaciated, Siddhartha awoke to the life-force in front of his eyes. The bullfrog's croaks halted, replaced by a single, infant-like scream. Above him, the golden full moon still hung in the brightening western sky.

That first spring morning, Siddhartha remained seated under the rich emerald green canopy. The welcoming space of liberation opened before him. A multitude of bugs flittered and crawled. The colony of glossy ibis and storks woke along the river's muddy banks. Night herons prepared for sleep, surrendering the day to the larger colonists. The egrets on the paddock croaked morning calls to the villagers, the wildlife, and livestock. The dawn light reflected through the dew on the grasses. A family of langur monkeys scrambled down from the tree to pick seeds and insects next to the still seated man.

Villagers started their day's labours. Word spread through the slow village about the man in the pipal grove. "Something happened earlier. Did you feel the earth tremble, or was it only my dream?" A curious few filed by the tree to investigate.

―――

The farmer and his wife made their way to the tree, proffering the morning rice and vegetables. A few neighbours trailed them — a woodcutter, a river-fisher, and a weaver-woman. The weaver carried two used, clean strips of cotton cloth. A small waist cloth would serve as his *langota*, cover his privates. The large piece, about two metres by three, would clothe the man's upper body and arms. While walking to the tree, she sang a song of spring.

Later, the farmer returned alone, but with full arms. He replaced the now-empty bowl from breakfast with mango and fermented coconut meat on a sal-tree leaf. At Siddhartha's feet, he spread gold marigolds and pink kachnar flowers. He also left a clean bowl. "This one's for fetchin' water."

Siddhartha, now robed in the weaver's offering, smiled, "Good sir, on your generous wife's fine grass mat, I engaged in a mighty struggle. I have won. I am free from angst, free from craving, and free of defilements. Both peasants and rulers of our country are slaves to tradition, ritual, and superstition."

The smile now gone, "The Brahmin priests are parasites, sucking human energy to their own gain, leaving behind poverty and ignorance. Alone, I comprehend suffering and the end of suffering. Other than the Great Earth herself, no one can teach me and I keep no students. I am now utterly alone."

No, the farmer thought, you are not alone. We are with you. If you hunger, we will feed you. If you teach, we will listen. If you lead, we will follow. Silently, the farmer pressed his palms together, bowed and left the man and his tree, remembering he needed to check the sex of the newborn kid.

## The vow under the tree

Siddhartha solved the puzzle that tormented him since youth, to find a way of liberation and kindness when the only certainty is death. Freedom, the stuff of Buddha-ness, is in each moment. Each moment carries the uncertainty of passing. Each moment carries the possibility of creativity. He became free now to express the dizzying kaleidoscopic blossoming of the moment. Each moment belongs to us all.

He remained under the tree; his quest accomplished. He'd found meaning and purpose, but they lay waiting, far from finished. The power of the life-force stirred within his deprived body. A new challenge lay ahead. The value he found lay within every person. It was not his possession. The life-force belonged equally to all living beings, to the universe itself. Everyone, high or low, wise or foolish, virtuous or evil, can free themselves of the constraints of anger, delusion, greed. Everyone is capable of the same enlightenment.

Mara, ever present, the unkillable, tried one last roll of the die:

"You won, Lord Buddha. You attained the unattainable, achieved what no one else has achieved, awakened to what no one else can realize. Go carefully, now, O Awakened One. Speak loosely of what can not be spoken, and you will confuse others. You will hurt those you seek to help. Proceed with great caution.

"You won, defeated even me, the undefeatable. Celebrate. You are done. Go home now. Your wife and precious son await. Your jealous cousin, Devadatta, awaits as well, lurking lustfully by your bed chamber. Consider, now, those close to you, those you care about most."

For the first time in a great while, Siddhartha thought of Yasodhara. He felt not the love and possessiveness of a husband, but trust and equality. Without sentimentality or regret, he recognized the woman he left behind, the teen-aged girl who chose him. As he now knew himself, he knew her. She was, in every way, his equal. The years and miles did not separate them. He thought of the milkmaid, the captain, the five ascetics, of all those who'd helped him. He must go forward, repay their favour.

"Nay, Lord Mara, I am not Buddha, not yet, not as long as this wonder remains unspoken. My awakening is meaningless while others remain asleep. Your role in this story continues.

"I will not go back. Instead, you will come with me, attend to me. Like the jester to a prince, like the shadow to a form, like the sword to a warrior, you will march by my side to the unknown. Even you, brother Devil King, share in this wonder. As once we shared the womb, we will go forth together.

"Somewhere in this land of sorrow, you and I will find those with little dust covering their sleepy eyes. I will teach them. Then, and only then, I will be Buddha. First, we go west to Baranasi, where my five ascetic companions head."

The question he faced, would face for his remaining forty years, was how others could experience their own awakening. What words would he find to explain what can not be explained? Like an inner whirlpool, his life-force swirled. The energy stirred him to a new purpose. He refused now to escape himself. He remained his fate.

A great vow welled forth. He would not stay silent. Out of his mouth poured the voice of life-force: "Living beings are numberless; I will save them all. All people will equally experience this enlightenment. Awakening is the fate of all living beings, and in this I take my vow."

## Arpeggio of joy

Now ready table and chairs prepared for guests. The table is set. Invitations sent. Come as you are, however wounded and scarred, however faint the hopes or shaky the intention. Seats wait, enough for the courageous and the despairing, the disappointed and the loving.

I take my place at the table. There's plenty of room here. Welcome.

Siddhartha's triumph can be replicated in this ambivalent, perilous moment. We can emulate his diligence, if not his practice, his vow to fight for other's well-being. We too can choose to face reality as it is, not as we'd like it to be. We can still recall our hidden promise.

Then, behold! Creativity inevitably emerges from daily effort. Our environment responds like an echo to our raucous shout. The joy of life-force rises from within.

Life-force surges. In the ebb and the flow, the crest and the trough. In the blooming and withering away. In the body, each atom vibrates to the eccentric dance of galaxies. In the microcosm that is us, formed of star-stuff, life-force swells in continuous co-creation, the divine embrace of self and environment.

When I view our precious world as it is, and all us fragile beings as we are, I see joy.

Joy the grin, curving lips breaking out and up.

Joy the laugh, the shiver not the joke.

Joy the shout.

Life-force. A joyous breath in, a single rotation of the Earth, one pirouette of Mother Earth's glorious dance 'round her sun. She rotates and we rise to welcome her day.

Bellies fill with the lusty inhalation of her morning. In the predawn fog of the Pacific Coast, the relentless rumble of oceanic tides pulse up and down in a rapturous duet of moon and water. Out of the deep come roars of Poseidon's timpani and tubas calling the tasks of the day:

This day, change a diaper, stir soup, study school books, create beauty, cultivate soil, grow the treasures of the heart. In the diligence that's due the day, through glistening sweat and occasional sob, each modest task clears a path to joy.

Earth turns to midday. A poem captures the fleeting moment. A pencil sketches an ant on a leaf on a branch in a grove. Across oceans and deserts, our hearts beat with another — each beat nurturing, elevating the other. Speak words of kindness; pat a shoulder, lend a hand. Give directions to a stranger. Hear their story. Loneliness turns to solitude, into a moment of solidarity.

Just as Mara ever returned to attack Siddhartha, our fear, doubt, and self-loathing still lurk in ambush. Today, too, an emphatic, decisive battle ensues. The planet turns. Sable Island mares nicker to their nursing foals under the pale yellow-green shimmering curtain of Northern Lights.

From the belly, the breath erupts in voice, vibrating a mantra of devotion. From the belly, creation guides worn fingers; life-force energizes tired muscles. In the Australian evening, a thousand hours of rehearsal and rigour arrive at the hall. The maestro pulses her curving rosewood baton. A violin's Bosnian maple and spruce turned and tuned into a smiling scroll. Strings in perfect fifths and the guts of the bow echo through the Sydney orchestra, into the packed hall and out to the encircling skies. And the audience, oh yes, the rapt audience raises the hall, as the enchanted chorus cheers an ode to joy.

Sing the day fulfilled. The vibration of that single breath reverberates across continents. Night falls over home, East Africa. The Lord of the Serengeti, wild mane matted in mud, scarred and weathered, lifts from his hindquarters and gazes at the smear of his revolving Milky Way in the cloudless night. From his belly comes a roar stirring woods and grass and sky for miles.

The vibrant joy of life-force thunders through joined voices, the beat of four hands on one drum, a teacher's embrace. A tree in India extends roots ever deeper and leaves ever fuller, and a prison somewhere is bulldozed into dust.

Here is the life-force, in our bodies and out, our breath rising and falling, our heart's percussion, and our gut's courage. Not the singer, nor the song, nor the chords, but joy's vibrant crescendo and the ever, ever diminuendo of the fading exhale.

This place, this circumstance — our apartment, hospital bed, the prow of a ferry, under a tree, or even in prison — here is where joy is reclaimed. You, dear reader, and I have arrived at this breath. Wherever we are and however we got here, now here.

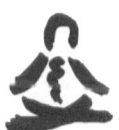

# PART THREE
# AWAKENINGS

> have the courage to not be clever
> the audacity to not use tricks
> to forget everything learned
> and honour my teachers
> with shy creation

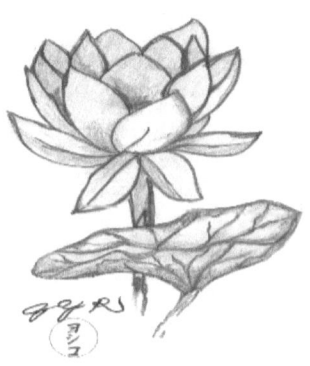

# wait with me

like the snail inside the lettuce,
like the water for the boil,
like the patient for the doctor,
and the one left behind,
wait with me.
For the light will surely change
if you wait with me
like the upbeat to this song,
I'll show you how.


Wait with me
like the cake inside the oven,
like the paper for the ink,
like patience for their virtues,
wait with me
For the moon will surely rise
like the upbeat to this song
I'll show you how.

Like the trigger for the finger,
and secrets for their shaming,
like roots for their blossoms,
like the best yet to come
wait with me.


Are you waiting for a call?
Wait with me.
Like the wine inside the barrel,
like the mirror for the razer,
like the masked executioner,
like the dream awaits the dawn,
wait with me.


For the play will soon be starting
and my seat is crying empty
and the line will soon be ending
like *dal segno* and this *finé*,
If you can wait with me
I'll show you how.

# Mom and Dad

RECENTLY I LEARNED A fairly elementary reproductive fact: A woman is born with a set number of ova. No more are created over her lifetime. Female babies carry all the eggs from their birth day. Inside my Mom when she was still a newborn is the ovum that Dad would fertilize, that became me.

In fact, the day before their birth, in utero, the female fetus also carries the eggs. Irene inside Emma, Peter, Stephen, and Keith inside Irene, three generations bound in a single body, one system. My family system goes beyond the related folks around now, goes back to those I never met. Their experiences affect me, in unseen yet real ways.

## Mom, San Francisco, 1930s–40s

Mom, her mother Emma, and her father, Joe, lived all over San Francisco. She recalled apartments they'd stayed in less than a month. They moved ahead of debt collectors, uncharitable landladies, and priests.

No one needed to tell Mom, "you're unwanted," but they concocted new ways to remind her. Emma, the daughter of Hungarian royalty, told Mom, "Any man in California could have been mine if you hadn't come along." Nobody needed to post a sign on the fridge: once she walked and talked, Mom cared for herself and the fragile bloom, Emma, and the thirsty ivy, Joe. Unwanted, but constantly in demand.

According to family lore, a girl in a convent became pregnant, had a daughter. The church excommunicated Joe. Mom reminisced about how every year the priests tracked Joe Manning down to remind him of his sin — "You stole Christ's wife." Despite the excommunication, Mom, a good Catholic girl, learned her catechism. That's what proper Hungarian royalty did.

Murky thing, excommunication — they boot you out, let you go, but keep holding on. Catholics tell me now this is not how excommunication actually works. Apologies. My telling here is consistent with how the family told it. And you know family stories. *Catholic Answers* magazine says that excommunication is a remedial penalty to correct misbehaviour. Between 1917 and 1983, excommunication included being excluded from the Church.[49]

## Dad, New York, 1944

On Friday the 29th, the last day of Chanukah, Ira packed a sandwich in a paper bag and told his mother that he'd be gone the entire day. The 2 line carried him from the Bronx into Manhattan, then the Fulton Street train out to Queens. While on the train, he wrote a few notes with a pencil in his notepad and pondered what to say. From the 80 Street station, he strolled eight minutes to the Acacia Cemetery. After inquiring at the office, he located his father's grave.

Ira spent a pleasant hour wandering around the orderly cemetery and the adjoining park. Acacia, an old Jewish cemetery, had graves going back to the eighteenth century. He wandered from grave to grave, reading the names and dates, unable to read the Hebrew epitaphs, curious about the buried.

Shalom, father. I've never done this. Spoken to a grave. What is the proper way? Anyway, fascism is threatening the entire world. Soon I'll be joining the Navy, the US Navy, so I thought I should visit you, if I don't come back. I didn't tell Mother I'd be coming here, but certainly she'd be happy. I am not religious, so won't be praying. Are you, I mean, were you religious? Were you agnostic? I've been told so little about you. Were you a kind man? Happy? Did you enjoy music, the opera, as much as Mother? Mother hasn't told much, and my brothers say they don't remember you. Thanks to you, Mother had an excellent start. And, well, you can appreciate how bright she is; she invested well, blue-chip, so we have been looked after. Thank you, father, for being my father. I wish I knew you, but wishing takes the same time as planning. I am going to help plan a new world after this war ends.

## Mom and Dad, San Francisco, 1944–1945

After the war, in late 1945, Irene took Commander Ira Miles Robinson, USN, home to meet the Hungarian royal family. Big family dinner. Ever since they heard that "Irene captured a Jew," they'd been abuzz.

Days before the dinner, Irene and Emma lunched on a downtown San Francisco restaurant patio. A short, overweight, balding man strolled by their table. Emma spotted her opening: "Your Jew fiancé will resemble him in a few years. But he will always be a good provider. They hoard all the money hidden in gold."

Irene ignored the bait. No need to talk back. She propped up straighter, filling her lungs with the Pacific air. Regular people united to beat back fascism. A new world approached. Ira cared, a man for the times, intelligent, progressive.

"At the dinner, try to keep up a good front, Irene. You'll need the support when your back breaks."

## The family dinner, San Francisco, CA, December 1945

Every family has its stories, mythology. Our family mythology shattered at a dinner table in late 1945. Grandma, the princess, hosted the pre-wedding dinner. Irene's Uncle Bud and Ira dressed in full ceremony uniforms, both still on active duty.

In 1940, the year before Pearl Harbor, Buddy volunteered for the US Army, two years under-aged. His mother, the princess, gave permission for Bud to enlist at nineteen.

At the dinner, Buddy and Ira hit it off. Both served at the Leyte Gulf Battle, considered the largest Naval battle in history. Buddy said: "I was a medical tech for quite a while, but I ended up a litter bearer when we invaded Leyte. I went in a volunteer; came out a pacifist."

Ira told Buddy about witnessing Hiroshima's devastation. "These weapons must never be used again." Both hated war; both hated fascism more.

Bud had five years of family news to catch up on. His mother's letters told him Irene had stayed at their house from time to time. He worried about Irene, three years younger than him, so tough and so fragile. But talking with Ira eased Bud's concerns for her well-being.

"What are your plans?" Buddy asked.

"After the wedding, hitchhike around the country; then to Chicago. Ira will take his masters in economics there. Then, he plans to do his doctorate in planning — urban and regional planning."

The princess: "Oh, you are marrying an architect. That is a respectable pursuit."

Irene held back their real motivations: a revolution approached. It would be messy and afterwards would need cleaning up. She and Ira would prepare for the mess and help plan the society to emerge after.

As the evening continued, out came the antisemitism with the booze. "Oh, yes, education is so important to you people." And the jokes. Jokes about Jews setting fire to their own businesses for insurance money, "Jewish lightning, ha ha ha." Jokes about bankers, about the Rothschilds.

Finally, Uncle Bud had enough. "I wish everybody would cut it out, since we are all Jewish."

Uh, no. What? How could we be Jewish?

---

Persecution of Hungarian Jewry increased in the years before the Holocaust. Some Hungarian Jews took desperate measures to protect themselves. They destroyed their histories and identity.

Mom's family rejected their heritage for self-protection and converted to Christianity. Eventually, they forgot their past, becoming antisemitic. Raised a Catholic in an antisemitic environment, Mom heard no hint of her true heritage. Even so, throughout her life, she carried the previous generation's trauma of self rejection. To save themselves, Hungarian Jewry hid. My forebears hid so well, they lost themselves.

## Pioneer House Care Home, Sacramento, 1989

Decades later, Mom and I bid Emma goodbye, her tiny frame propped up in an oversized hospital bed. Attendants raised the bed to its maximum height.

Mom's slightly less tiny body climbed onto the bed, kneeling next to her mother. What are you doing, Ma? Would she strangle Emma to be sure this meant goodbye?

For a minute, Mom put aside her crusty, chain smoking, Jameson sipping, Shakespeare quoting, tough girl exterior. And she put aside the helpless little girl forced to care for the helpless adult who was supposed to care for her. Mom kneeled on the bed next to Emma. For a minute Mom became an adult woman, caring with empathy and love for another woman.

"C'mon Momma, if a girl's going out, she's gotta be ready." Mom pulled lipstick from her purse and precisely drew Emma's lips, adjusting with a wet tissue. Then she applied rouge carefully to her mother's cheeks. Mom had her compact out and turned the mirror so Emma saw herself.

I stood at the bedside, witness to a miracle. My eyes welled with tears of grief and pride. Mom shimmied off the bed, her usual wet eyes dry.

"I know a decent fish and chips place, ol' Keith. My dime."

## A garden in Japan, Kyoto, Spring 1990

A few months after Emma passed, I took Mom to Japan. We toured the temples and their gardens in Kyoto, her lifelong dream. She scrutinized the gardeners, women minutely tending the plants. "See what they are doing, Keith? They separate the mosses, one species from the other, the good moss from the bad. The spring moss spreads rusty yellow, not yet turned fully green. The others showed dark, almost purple."

I appreciated the beauty, but to my eye, all the moss appeared the same. "Mom, something not mentioned in the tourist pamphlets: Until about a hundred-fifty years ago, they forbid women from entering these temples' grounds, even as gardeners. The priests considered women defiled and a woman's presence would pollute these holy sites."

---

At the famous rock garden at Ryoanji Temple, Mom wept on the veranda. Fifteen rocks and gravel in a rectangular space form the UNESCO World Heritage site, a garden without blooms or water.

Mom may have interpreted the garden as an enlightenment symbol, or a pinnacle of human achievement. Perhaps she attained her highest aspirations, her own garden sanctuary. Mom blossomed there, planted on the edge of a garden without flowers.

She found the garden for her younger self, forbidden to be a child. The little girl who set her mother's hair in rollers and put her mother to bed. Then dove into the old San Francisco night to fetch her father from behind the Shamrock Tavern. The hopes fulfilled of a tormented girl who found solace in plants and gardens. Finally, nothing had been wasted. For a moment I witnessed Mom whole.

## The search for our family, 2004

One day when I got home from work, Yoshiko said, "Your Uncle Bud phoned."

"Buddy? From Hawai'i?"

"He's found your family. He is organising a gathering in California."

"That's fantastic. Any details? Did you talk to him? He's a good guy."

"He asked about my Mommy and Daddy, their lives in Manchuria and Siberia. According to Bud, I should write my family history, for the sake of the future."

This was new. "Great idea. Can I help?"

"No." Yoshiko said, "I'm not writing anything."

Buddy buried the royalty myth way back at the family dinner in 1945. In the early 2000s, he had retired and was dying of prostate cancer. As his last task, he set to root out who we were, if not Hungarian royalty. "Know from whence you came. If you know whence you came, there is really no limit to where you can go," James Baldwin wrote.[50] Uncle Bud believed we owe it to the future to understand our past. For Buddy, finding our roots became his life's work, not a retirement hobby. He didn't search out of curiosity, but an all-consuming longing. Finding his roots, who survived, who endured, who remained, equalled finding himself. He scoured online genealogy sites. Hobbled by a merciless disease, Buddy flew to Hungary, explored graveyards, and hired a private detective.

Meanwhile, in Israel, two elderly brothers wondered if anyone survived of their family. To their knowledge, everyone died in the Holocaust. The younger one browsed the Internet. He came across Buddy. Buddy found them. They worked together and uncovered others in Italy, the US, Australia, Canada.

## The Jonas family meets

Families hold reunions. We celebrated a union. Around sixty of our new family gathered at a hotel in San Mateo, California. Our daughters, Erica and Andrea, and I attended. People came who'd accepted life without family. Some expected to exit this world believing they were alone. Artists and bakers and academics.

It turns out our family name was Jonas, like Jonah, the prophet. And like Jonah, sixty complete strangers came out from the whale's dark belly of solitude into the light of instant familial love and acceptance.

Together, the family watched the 1999 film *Sunshine*. *Sunshine* tells the story of three generations of a Hungarian Jewish family through empire, Nazis, and communism. The horrors that the family suffered were not inflicted by Germans or foreigners, but by fellow Hungarians they lived beside. *Sunshine* proved painful to view. The film portrayed horrific violence, but also internal violence. In their failed efforts to belong, to assimilate, to contribute to their own country, the family committed a kind of group identity suicide.

The three hour film conveyed the reality of intergenerational trauma. Several of our family's elders could not handle watching. They huddled outside in the hotel hall. Other elderly family members stayed, "for the sake of the next generations," slumped in the back, quietly weeping.

Speakers presented papers on the Jonas family history. Uncle Bud distributed genealogical charts from his tireless research. Tears of joy and belonging shed. Speeches made and stories told. Pictures exchanged. Who we were.

For three days I came home, encountering a family I never knew but always had. My disconnected lifetime transformed by three days of love and acceptance.

Mom didn't attend, her health failing. I phoned, told her about the meeting, about her family that she never knew. Who we are; how hard Uncle Bud worked to locate and gather us; what a beautiful family we are. Within the year, we lost both her and Buddy.

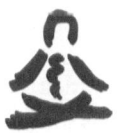

# The Hungry Ghost

### Candy in a bowl, Late 1960s

TWELVE YEARS OLD AND visiting family friends. It's a pleasant Southern California house. Clean, with cheerful mid-century modern furniture. Nobody there. A cast metal candy bowl decorated the teak coffee table. Left in the open and filled with candy, anyone could dig in, help themselves. Anyone could snatch all the candy. I froze. Nobody around to catch me.

At the time, the experience felt dreamlike, other-worldly, as if in slow-motion. I stared at the bowl through thick shimmering LA afternoon light blurring the room and the table.

Now the memory commands a three-dimensional solidity. The curved candy drops, round and right, each glinting from the afternoon sun through sheer curtains. The bite-sized, perfect spheres stacked in graceful symmetry. Each enticing drop invites, promises wholeness.

The clean teak coffee table is like an artefact from a superior civilization. Dust motes, streaming into the room in dustlight, carry messages: "Our confidence is quiet, fulfilled. For you, we leave furniture and candy." This impossible place shared its plenty too easily. Such largess. Such generosity and trust. Shameful.

Of course, I didn't steal any candy. Impossible. If I reached towards the bowl, my hand would pass into a different dimension, parallel and forbidden. I remained condemned to my side of the thin curtain, forever craving and soiled.

## Realm of the hungry ghosts

Among the mythical creatures I encountered in my Buddhist studies were the Preta, the hungry ghosts. The hungry ghosts bear huge, insatiable bellies and necks thin as needles. They scrounge for whatever waste they can consume. But once food reaches their desperate mouths, it explodes in fire and smoke. They spend ages in unsatisfied craving.

Perhaps "hungry ghost" is redundant. Every ghost is hungry, unsatisfied. Otherwise, why hang around old Victorian houses, abandoned cellars, in dreams and memories?

The Preta crave for the impossible, to rewind the clock on a lifetime's regrets. The hungry ghosts long for all they've lost and all they've tossed away. They lust and they aren't receiving. And, if they fulfill their desires, it's not enough, never enough.

---

Here we are on our blue planet of depleting resources, of such abundance. With not enough, with too much. What's to be done for us pitiful, hungry ghosts with our endless cravings, our semi-conscious consumption?

For some, gambling. Or alcohol. Or sex, shopping, drugs. For me, food. It has always been food.

My stomach hurts. Treat it. Feed it. Relieve pain by stuffing it. Filling it. If I love my guts, I feed them. Right?

Food is scarce. Devour now, or gone forever. And then?

After all, food is love. We feed whom we love. If they loved me, they'd feed me. Corollary: if I consume, I am loved.

People nibble half and toss away the rest. Disgusting. So shameful. Don't they maintain any decency? Don't waste food. Gobble it now. Quickly. Quickly.

Devour it before it wastes, before the full button clicks, before the shame kicks in, before anyone sees me.

## A mother disappears, India, ~409 BCE

One of the Buddha's disciples, the legends say, mastered the ancient magic arts. Kolita studied sorcery, spells and counterspells, divination, alchemy, and astrology. He became renowned as foremost in occult powers.

One day, Kolita's mother vanished. He searched everywhere, questioned everyone. His eyes took on a pained, watery gaze with deep circles underneath, his countenance grim and distracted. He panicked. Using occult powers of divination, he discovered she had fallen into the realm of the hungry spirits. Indeed, he actually peered into the spirit realm. There she suffered horribly, tortured by demons, starved. Kolita's misery and panic are familiar to all those with a loved one captured by craving. He used his magic to enter the spirit realm to feed his mother. But the food he offered her turned to fire, torching her mouth. Her desperate mouth lunged at the acrid smoke for nourishment. His poor, pitiful mother became a Preta, a hungry ghost. Her neck stretched needle-thin; her empty, grumbling belly, large as an elephant.

## Jetavana Monastery, Srāvastī, Kingdom of Kosala

During the monsoons, June through October, the Buddha stayed in a hut at the Jetavana (Jeta's Grove) Monastery, outside Srāvastī city. Today, the Archaeological Survey of India maintains the site's remains in present-day Uttar Pradesh.

During the Buddha's time, wealthy lay supporters built Jetavana in a grove of *madkam* butter trees and mango trees. Near his hut stood a pond for the Buddha to bathe. Besides the simple wood and brick hut, the complex held monk's dormitories, latrines, an auditorium, and dining hall. Outside the monastery proper, they constructed the nun's compound.

The Buddha's hut itself was the simplest structure, enough to provide protection from the elements. Inside lay a pallet for sleeping and a wooden dais for him to greet guests. The Buddha's possessions sat on the pallet — two spare robes, folded; two bowls, one for food and the other for washing; a razor, and a water strainer. Aromatic blossoms and incense fragrance filled the air. They called it the Scented Hut.

## A belly burning with passion, The Scented Hut

Kolita desperately sought a way to aid his suffering mother. He sought his mentor's advice.

Inside the Scented Hut's single room, mango wood pillars divided the modest, ordered space. Wide windows on all the walls allowed in soft light, diffused by adjustable lattice window coverings. Smoke from incense further diffused the light and discouraged hungry mosquitos. A sand layer and then cushions blanketed the packed dirt floor.

In the centre, the now elderly Buddha perched on a low dais. The boy who sat an elephant and wondered about roles and identity, the man who awoke under a fig tree, was now seventy. Kolita's master sat cross legged, slumped to the left, his arm on a wood prop, his back supported by a rough hemp bolster filled with beans.

Behind the dais, a pallet bed lay below a single shelf on the wall. Three or four jars for medicine sat on the shelf. For several months each year, the restless man who left family and home seeking liberation paused his wanderings and made this space home.

A medley of aromas filled Kolita's nose and head. Lay believers brought fragrant flowers daily to be strewn around the space or floated in bowls. On this day, the space overflowed. The proffered stems and blossoms backed up to line the path outside.

Acolytes maintained the hut. They tried to keep the ever-growing flower piles in order. Followers brought monsoon blooms in a continuous stream of balsam, hibiscus, and lotus. Their priority was to honour the sincerity of the donors. They sorted the growing piles of fresh and withered blooms, sending edible flowers to the kitchen. Others took medicinal flowers to the infirmary to be dried or distilled into elixirs.

But the space could become chaotic, with blooms in piles and people coming and going. The flowers piled and decomposing. Guests, kings and peasants, patrons and supplicants arrived for encouragement, negotiation, or debate.

At the centre sat a seventy-year-old. Here, he talked and guided and debated, laughed and occasionally admonished. Elsewhere in the complex, he practised, bathed, ate, and preached.

The bouquets, garlands, and buds invigorated the Buddha's home. To Kolita, they also evoked the mutual devotion between mentor and followers.

Kolita bowed. "Is the World-Honoured One well and at ease?"

"Ah, dear Maudgalyayana," the Buddha used Kolita's formal name, "I become frail and aged. Like a rickety cart, I am lashed together with supports. My body ages, as do all bodies. But my mind is clear, my heart is at ease, my belly continues to burn with passion for the salvation of all."

"Blessed One, your voice softens, but I still detect the lion's roar."

The Buddha chuckled. "Aye, and the old lion's paws still itch, even if two legs become three." Kolita noticed the bamboo cane by his mentor's side. "When the highways dry, Maudgalyayana, let's march on the great road. Let's sleep beneath the stars. We should stride the long path to Eagle Peak again. There I will speak words yet unspoken, words of interest to those yet to be born. The season for the lotus blossoming approaches."

Kolita sat upright on a mat at the dais foot. Tall, his head almost reached the height of the slumped Buddha's head. Next to Kolita, a disciple waited quietly to witness and put the Buddha's words to memory. To the Buddha's right, an acolyte stationed himself, also silent, with a water gourd and a fan, if the master required anything.

Although the others were present, Kolita felt alone with his mentor, in a shining golden home of trust and love and welcome. His dour countenance briefly softened. His face took on a child-like innocence, eager and sincere. A shared moment with his teacher.

But the compulsion proved too strong. Mother is in the realm of hungry spirits; don't waste time here. He squirmed on the mat. The moment of shared purpose passed. He chewed his lower lip. The chords on his neck protruded. From child-like to childish in a flash.

The Buddha broke the silence. "My heart is at ease, but I sense yours is troubled."

It came out in a rush: "Blessed One, help me. My dear mother suffers. She has become a desperate Preta, a Preta, Lord, tormented unceasingly. I beseech you, Lord, help save her." Saying the words gave rise to his own insatiable hunger.

He lost the moment of connection. The Buddha ceased being his beloved mentor, united in purpose. Instead, in that instant, he became to Kolita a saviour, a god to petition for favour and relieve his pain. He would attempt anything to save her, even lose himself.

"Saving your mother is the highest of filial piety, the source of virtue and humanity. Kolita, through practicing the way, you have become a sage of great order; yet you are unable to help your poor mother, who suffers horribly. Despite your praiseworthy efforts, you fail to rescue her, unable to repay the debt of kindness you owe her.

"Alone, Kolita, you can do nothing for your poor mother. All your skills, your life's achievements, will be in vain. Find your refuge in the community. You will only receive aid from the believer's community, from connection. Put your trust in people, not magic."

---

Kolita left the Scented Hut crushed, more distraught than ever. He wandered the grounds aimlessly. Of what use was all his training, his studies, if none helped to save his poor mother? Why be foremost in occult power if it were powerless? He couldn't stop himself. After all, this was his mother.

In the following days, he sought advice from sorcerers and necromancers. Somewhere, something must help. He no longer even remembered her from before. What kind of mother had she been? What did she so desperately crave?

Despite the Buddha's instruction, despite himself, he returned repeatedly to the realm of the Pretas. He couldn't quit. He longed to see if the demons continued to torment her. Did she consume anything today, even dung or rotten flesh? Beyond himself in grief, he compulsively employed his powers to gawk at her in the land of the Pretas, over and over. Everything worsened both their anguish. All his efforts turned to acrid smoke.

## Exploding food and burnt lips

Instead of committing himself to the community, Kolita became negligent, slackening in his duties. Saving his mother ate at his mind, distracting his prayers. He finished services quickly and used his powers to return to her in the spirit realm.

One day he realized he must care for himself. He bathed at the stone washing pool in the complex's south-east corner. He began to shave his head and beard. That's when he noticed his stretched neck. He peered down at his stomach. His belly ballooned.

"I will eat well at the daily meal. The rule that monks consume a single meal a day seems unreasonable, especially for a tall chap like me."

After bathing, Kolita headed to the meal hall. Others glanced at him, doing double takes at his odd appearance. Famished, he loaded his bowl with rice, lentils, and squash. While he plopped into a corner, he skimmed through his pre-meal prayer. He scooped a handful from the bowl to his mouth.

The food exploded in fire and smoke. His food ignited, scorching his fingers and mouth.

Now everyone in the hall stared. Before their astonished eyes, Kolita was becoming a Preta, enslaved to his talents and self-image. He screamed in pain and scanned the hall for water, for any help. Only one person moved.

An elderly woman raced across the dirt floor of the hall. Her golden moon eyes fixed like a predator's on Kolita. She moved on the toes and balls of her unclad feet with the agility of a young lioness, not of a woman in her seventieth year.

Kolita cowered, a cornered antelope. She spoke, her voice resounding regally, at once caring and reproaching.

"You are a mighty Bodhisattva, a noble warrior of liberation. You have even become a Preta yourself to save the Hungry Ghost. Rejoice. The time has arrived to fulfil your mission. Expand your petty cravings into determination to spread the dharma."

"I can't... My mouth... I can't. I hurt. My mother... I must see to my mother. Improper this... a monk speaking directly with a woman."

She leaned closer. Standing, she was eye to eye with the seated, cowering man. Her wrinkled, age-spotted face filled his view.

Would she strike him, bite him, rip him with her claws?

"Improper? You fear your foolish words will seed this old shrivelled womb? Be more afraid of what awaits neglecting your life's purpose. That slight tinge on your lips is a firefly's spark compared to hell's inferno in your future."

"I... I... it's injured... burned... "

"What did our mentor instruct you? Speak now."

He got the words out. "The community. The Blessed One taught to seek salvation in the community."

"Did he?" The old woman paused, stepped back, no longer eye to eye, thinking. "I see. He's right. Come with me."

## A story of the Buddha's ex-wife

The woman was none other than Yasodhara, the Buddha's ex-wife. The thirteen-year-old girl who chose Siddhartha was here. How she transformed from an abandoned single mother to become a ferocious disciple, she will shortly tell.

Yasodhara took Kolita to call on members of the community of believers. They made a curious sight: the tall, solemn monk, his blistered mouth wrapped in poultice, trailing the diminutive elderly woman.

The people they met shared their experiences in life and in faith. Each told the worry or suffering that led them to the dharma. Many told of losing a loved one; others, tales of abuse they suffered; some of losing homes to natural disaster or human cruelty. Others suffered from crippling disease or deformity. All life's miseries.

The women told horrific stories of masters treating them like livestock. They shared poignant tragedies of lost children, lost lovers, and lost spouses. He listened closely to the mothers' stories, commiserating silently.

For the first time, he considered the Buddha's own mother, who passed away shortly after childbirth. Have we all lost the woman who carried us, whose belly we shared? As his ears heard, his heart moved.

Once the burn on his lips healed, Kolita shared his story with those they met. He told of his mother's disappearance, his desperate search, and finding her as a Preta. He had yet to determine what craving compromised her. How he became a slave to fixing what none could repair. But he refused to abandon the woman who carried him for nine months and fed him at her breast. Both the women and men listened to his tale.

As he shared his story, his awareness of his mother grew, of what she did for him. Even if she was a Preta, an addicted slave to craving, for nine months she'd been present for him, existed *for* him in a way no other human being could. By heeding his fellow's experiences and by honestly sharing his own, he cherished what his mother meant to him, what motherhood means.

The mothers he met wanted their children to be healthy, to live fulfilled lives. They wanted their children to be emotionally and spiritually strong and to find a purpose. Could this be what his mother craved? Was she agonising for him?

Engaged in this deep dialogue, listening and being heard, his heart both broke and opened. Something was happening to him.

---

Yasodhara shared her story — her indescribable grief and humiliation at Siddhartha's abandonment. For six years, she longed desperately and obsessively searched for him, raising their son alone. After receiving news of his awakening, his quest realized, she became his disciple. She admitted to her longing, her anguished, impossible longing to alter how things were into how she wanted them to be. How she healed through engaging in daily life. How she realized enlightenment, not through solitary meditation, but through solidarity.

## Three generations of struggle and resilience

One evening, Kolita and Yasodhara called on a poor family at their home. A heartfelt discussion opened with a simple recitation together:

We take refuge in the Buddha.
We take refuge in the Dharma.
We take refuge in the Community.

Then Kolita stood and recited thrice by himself:

I take refuge in the Community.
I take refuge in the Community.
I take refuge in the Community.

He lowered himself onto a mat on the packed dirt floor. Grandfather welcomed the two, speaking in a simple local Pali dialect, not in the rough language of the lower castes. At first the men spoke in turn, then the women. Three generations talked of crops and weather and sickness and children. Soon they cross-talked and back-talked, chortling and chattering. A mother in her mid-teens attended silently while her newborn suckled noisily. In a corner of the home, hens clucked on their indoor roost. In another corner, three youngsters played jacks with flat rocks. From time to time, they glanced up at Yasodhara while ignoring their parents and the dour, gangly monk.

Kolita glanced at the elderly nun in the single oil lamp's light. Her pale skin shone like buffed brass. Gazing into her keen, aged eyes, he imagined seeing his own lost mother. She smiled contentedly, whole, no longer broken by craving. For a moment, this was not a family talking *about* the Buddha's teachings. For a moment, their talk *became* the Buddha's teachings. They spoke from their hearts and guts and head. Their caring words back and forth and the sound rising and falling, and the cadence and vibration formed a kind of sutra, reverberating in the air.

Yasodhara told her story in the same local dialect as Grandfather. The family and Kolita listened intently. "We married after I turned sixteen. I loved Siddhartha so, my prince on Earth and my sun in the Heavens. His mind was troubled, his heart restless. We talked for hours. He could speak with me, just us two. 'Why do we suffer? Is there any person, any being, who does not suffer? Is there a key to unlocking this prison of living, suffering, dying? What is the point of our actions, our belongings, our vanities?' Over and over he questioned. He questioned his tutors, seniors, farmers, cobblers, kitchen maids."

Her voice echoed through the home, measured and determined. Both her words and their sound resonated within the listeners.

She continued. "I thought our love, my love, would ease his troubles. I thought if I loved him truly, I'd free him from his questions. Together, we two would be enough to resolve his doubts. To keep such a man gave me pride, so different from other men. Ah, my foolish pride, my vanity destined me to suffer. How do I possess a man who does not believe in possessions?"

The father gently interrupted, "Elder Sister, we heard the family's privilege protected him from the world's sufferings. We heard he encountered four people who showed life's misery: a sick person, an elder, a corpse, and a holy man. These meetings motivated him to set forth and seek freedom from suffering."

"Admittedly I've heard such stories, but not from his mouth. My husband inquired about every family in our clan, endlessly curious about people and the world. We shared the belief that every person, high or low, should live a fulfilling life. Suffering is certain. He became obsessed with discovering a virtuous way to live when the only certainty is passing."

Yasodhara spread her thin palm toward the playing children and listening seniors. "He inquired about the children and their studies. He'd say, 'Every Shakya boy and every girl, high or low, must learn propriety from an *acharya* teacher.' He inquired into the elders' health and their comfort. His father trained him for leadership, how to count the stores of grain, livestock, and the measure of the yearly floods. Every day he observed sickness, ageing, and death. Every day he probed sickness, ageing, and death.

"As for holy men, he met many who called themselves holy. He quizzed them, listened, and argued. Oh, he argued. 'No merit is gained from your animal sacrifices. One death will never result in reward to another. What god or devil created this miserable world? What is the value of teaching paradise after death if today people only experience craving and suffering?'

"I witnessed him harangue the holy Brahmins. 'You declare the castes are the natural order. Men above women. Priests above all. In the far west, the Yonans accommodate only two castes, citizens and slaves. Is nature different in the west?'

"He spoke of leaving, to be sure. It was no surprise. As his doubts grew, his resolve to uncover answers also grew. His fixation terrified me. My mind and heart were at war. I held the same questions as he: how to help our suffering people? Was life to be the empty repetition of duty and ritual? I did everything to love him more, fulfill my duties as his wife.

"Years passed, and he planted his seed in me. I thought, this will bind him to me. His child will bring him peace. If the two of us are not enough to settle his mind, a family will. Ah, a foolish child I remained. Being with a child only made him think more of others, of the future generations to come. 'Are all beings destined to suffer? There must be a way to freedom. I must locate it.'

"I'd lost him. He had never been mine to lose. Still, his leaving devastated me beyond my imagination. He abandoned us to renounce cravings, to sever ties that became chains. Why couldn't I love him enough? A thousand times, I questioned myself. I queried the gods. For six years, I anguished. I prayed to every god. He did not come home. I cursed every god. I cursed him for not returning to my questions. He did not return.

"As Rahula grew, he naturally inquired, 'Where is father?' My nights passed sleeplessly. If he came home while I slept, he might leave again. Where was he? Would he come back to his country? I queried every messenger, every traveller on the Great Northern Road.

"He did not return, but the rumours did. Word spread that he wandered in Magadha. He took up with a band of ascetics. Others claimed he'd become an evil bandit, preying on the innocent, or that he'd retreated north into the mountains, living with a monkey troop. The story arrived that he starved in the forests, a ruined, homeless hermit.

"He was gone. But I lived, raised our son, loved and served our clan. I loved, not selfishly to possess, but to nurture." She fixed Kolita directly in her gaze. "Love doesn't need be a chain imprisoning us in craving. Love is the needle pulling threads to bind wounds.

"He abandoned us, yes, but I refused to be forever the one left behind. Without him, I breathed. Clothed in joyous yellow, and white purity, I ate without him, danced with the seasons, and bled with the moon. As a mother and a Shakyan woman, I completed my duties wholeheartedly. In time, the chores of daily living, the kitchen, the field, gossiping with clanswomen, became a joy. Slowly I understood: his quest, wherever he was, wandering alone, became my quest with our people.

"Around six years later, other stories came from the east and south. A caravan captain reported people in Magadha spoke of a Buddha's emergence. Then others told similar stories: the World-Honoured One is come, they declared. Prithvi Mata, Mother Earth herself, quakes and dances. As these stories reached me, my mind calmed, less shaken. I cared about him, but obsession no longer ruled me.

"One afternoon, my man-servant came to me. 'A monk in saffron robes waits at the city gates, requesting the Lady of the Shakyas.'

"'Instruct the kitchen to prepare a simple meal befitting a holy man. After he is fed and bathed, bring him to me. Meanwhile, ensure Rahula is kept to his quarters. If this monk brings news of his father, I want my son to learn from my mouth.'"

The women listening to Yasodhara glanced at each other, nodding, yes, that is proper.

"Indeed, the monk brought news, not rumour. The quest was accomplished. My husband attained the supreme enlightenment. He taught in the Deer Park in Baranasi Forest. The monk said, 'The World-Honoured One teaches of suffering and suffering's end. The end of suffering lies on a middle path between self-indulgence and self-denial.'

"I told the monk, 'His liberation is my joy. Realizing his heart is calm gladdens my own.'

"I too became free. I felt the joy of liberation. He no longer was my husband. I decided then to follow him as my teacher. What he discovered in solitude, I would gain from connection. At that moment, I lost interest in becoming close to him as a wife, but to stride the path with others, as a woman."

Yasodhara's voice, packed with purpose, filled the home with purpose.

## The fire of lust lights the lamp of enlightenment

"It is now over forty years since the night he left me, our son, his home. He returned home once, after his enlightenment under the tree. Rahula had turned seven. We discussed the business of Rahula's inheritance. I spoke directly with the Buddha only that one time."

At that, the women shifted in their seats, their sarees rustling. A middle-aged woman raised a hand to her forehead. The statement surprised all, even Kolita. "Only once, Venerable Lady? But he is here, with us at Jeta's. I met him at the Scented Hut, pleading for my mother, the hungry ghost. We expect you to enjoy a special relationship with the Blessed One."

Several of the family nodded. Grandfather leaned his calloused body towards her. Yasodhara answered: "I am a single disciple. I do not need to encounter our mentor to follow or protect him, nor to teach others. Do not seek the wondrous dharma in a special place, a special relationship. The path is here, in this palace that is your home, in this family's kinship, in your very bodies."

Kolita had difficulty following. This complicated woman converted her unobtainable craving and obsession into connection and awakening. Cravings likewise consumed his mother. He likewise obsessed. Could it be that our desires were not the root of suffering but could be turned towards freedom? He struggled even to form the question.

"Venerable Lady, your longing, your desire — you did not extinguish it?"

"Nay, dear friend. As impossible as it was to satisfy my longings, they were impossible to extinguish."

The old woman took a deep inhale and gazed intently at each family member in turn. When she got to Grandfather, he bowed to kiss her feet, showing his deepest reverence. Before his lips touched, she grasped his face, gently guiding it to her own. Grandfather and the Buddha's wife sat face to face, gap-toothed to wrinkled grin, their eyes and chuckles meeting. She stroked his wrinkles as if smoothing creased fabric.

She released him. Both still smiled, and stopped laughing. She pulled back, her chest opened, heart lifting to the ceiling. From her mouth roared the thunder of the lioness queen:

"The lotus blossoms from the mud. The needle must puncture for the thread to bind. In the same way, your ignorance will become wisdom. Your sufferings will liberate your creativity. And your lusts will fire enlightenment's lamp."

---

After farewells to the family, the two ambled through the evening back to Jeta's. Leaving Yasodhara at the women's quarters, he bowed deeply to her parting figure.

He lurked at the gates, hovering alone in his thoughts. Curious, here I long to save my mother and I've never openly spoken with any woman. Never truly gave attention to them, never fully shared. In Yasodhara's company, Kolita's own vision expanded. Awakening belonged not to one man alone beneath a tree. All men and women and children under roofs or trees or sky can enjoy the freedom to live fulfilling, awakened lives.

As he lingered at the gate alone, his mentor's words came to mind: "my belly still burns with passion for the salvation of all." The question Kolita now faced, and would face for the rest of his days: how to shift his hunger towards compassion? How could he support his mentor to lead people to their liberation? He bowed again to the shadow where the old woman melted away. Finally, Kolita headed back to the ashram.

# THE HUNGRY GHOST

The Buddha fulfilled his wish to tramp the highways with Kolita. Later, after the roads dried, the community marched five hundred kilometres south and east. On an outcrop of stones in Magadha called Eagle Peak, the Buddha taught the Lotus Sutra. In the Lotus, he predicted Kolita's enlightenment. To Kolita, this prediction became "like sweet dew bathing me, washing away fever and imparting coolness. Joy and peace of mind will quickly be mine."[51]

According to legends, Kolita's efforts even saved his mother. They say she left the hungry spirit realm and ascended to heaven. To this day, many Asian countries still honour Kolita's achievement of saving his mother. On the fifteenth day of the seventh month, by the lunar calendar, Hungry Spirit festivals celebrate and honour the deceased.[52]

# Lean Forward

Into emptiness
Into the nameless
Forward to the purple ocean,
to the borders of space
Go forward to your home.

Standing at a precipice before the purple sea,
Lean forward.
Lean forward toward that darkness
Lean forward to the slippery rocks,
to the silver fat fish,
to the scurrilous tidepool rodents.

Perched on a ledge above the pregnant sea and
under the endless sky,
Lean up to the clockwork heavens to Saturn's hexagon,
the sacred transformational geometry of sky and self.

With you between sky and sea:
Mermen, sirens, descendants of Abraham sailing for Australia on a dilapidated ship.

Not a fevered vision,
no wistful ideals,
the hollow platitudes spent;
Now, lean forward.

# LEAN FORWARD

Embrace the uncertainty of the axe-king dealing tarot.
Each step out the front door, a commitment.
Each step an act of trust.

Lean into fragility.
Your beliefs are constructs held in place by brittle brown
firmament-thin fascia reflecting in a drop of dew.
Discard them.

                                              Lean down to the earth:
                          the carrots bring messages from the subsoil.
                 Witness the singular wonder of a moist grain of rice.

                                         Lean forward one final time
                                            Your day when all debt,
            all betrayal, resentments, and grudges will vanish,
                                 playing taps into the darkness,
                                     and find your creation,
                                             your renewal.

Do not return.
Do not anticipate outcomes — energy, creativity, the void.
Lean forward.
Forward.

# Stephen's Story

## Magic at a diner, Vancouver, 1959

AROUND FIVE YEARS OLD. Stephen, six or seven. A rare family meal out, the five of us crammed into a booth on padded bench seats, waiting for the server to approach and take Dad's order for our lunch. Mom and Dad faced us boys across the formica table. Stephen stared out the window, and Peter read a menu. Not sure why Peter had a menu, Dad will order for us. Sandwiched between them, I play with a spoon, staring into its polished reflection.

Funny, the things that stick in memory. All these years, chrome and shiny steel and the deep-fat fryer smell. Chrome trimmed the long counter like a car bumper. Steel shone from the oversized percolator and stainless cabinets behind the counter.

Another young family perched in a corner opposite us. Their toddler cried. The parents tried to hush it, but the crying continued. Normal people with a bawling baby. With Peter in my way, I can't see the baby.

Dad jabbed his pipe in the air. "Feh. I told you, we should have packed a lunch. Overpriced, slow service, and now a wailing baby. I'm not made of gelt, Irene."

Dad's outburst got Stephen's attention. He sat up, turned towards the crying. Stephen raised himself, twisting on the bench to see.

The crying continued. Mom tried to settle Dad, "Ira . . . Robbie . . ." putting a hand on his elbow. His arm recoiled. I lowered my head, stared down at my fingers tracing the table's chrome trim curves. This goes bad, I hide beneath the table. I hoped Mr Magoo-Dad wouldn't speak to the server. Bring the food fast, please, get this over. I toyed with my spoon, flipping it over, everybody reflected in the bowl. Turning the spoon over and over. Too young for the words concave and convex, I gazed into the shiny mirror, into another world.

Peter, his chin raised, lips parted, lowered his menu, caught Dad's gaze: "Babies cry, father. You did. I did."

Stephen stood, one hand on my shoulder. Let's do this. Dad ordered him to sit. Stephen ignored Dad, without a word, squeezed past me, past the glass sugar dispenser with a chrome lid, past our legs, past Pete's obstructing elbow. He marched over to the family, his back straight. Over to the little kid. I only made out Stephen's back in the other family's clump. Peter blocked my view of what Stephen said or did, but it should have been me. As the youngest, nearest to a toddler, it should have been me.

In seconds, Stephen finished. The crying stopped. The toddler cooed.

Stephen had magic.

## Envy, California, 1960s

Stephen, the problem child, began drinking and smoking from around nine or ten. He became sexually active from ten or eleven (how physically possible is beyond my ken). Kicked out of schools and in trouble with the law.

Mom and Dad struggled to find him support. They sent him to special schools and to therapists and programs and who knows what.

Charismatic, fiercely independent and self-contained, he forcefully persisted in being himself. Stephen mirrored all I wasn't — strong, stubborn, capable.

At home, he practised wrestling holds and throws on me — the full nelson, the half-nelson, and the body slam. He hid my homework and stole my allowance, humiliated me for my pathetic efforts to attract girls and all the things big brothers do. But outside the house, he championed me. He taught me to ride a bike, how to deliver newspapers. He took me to the donut shop that gave kids the broken pieces if we rode our bikes there early enough, before they opened. At the Fun House, he showed me where to perch on the spinning disk so I'd stay on the longest and win a prize. How loud he cheered for me, if I won a prize. And outside he stuck up for me, his kid brother, the magician's assistant. Keith will outsmart you guys. Keith throws a ball harder, faster, farther. When I explored too deep into the Presidio, lost in myself, darkness descending, Stephen would find me and deliver me home.

Women loved him and took him home. Later, he taught me to roll joints and tried to teach me how to attract girls. I envied Stephen all his strengths, his refusal to follow the rules. He didn't need to question or doubt his identity or wonder if he fit. But I most envied his ability to be cruel. He'd be so shamelessly cruel. I didn't wish to be, but envied him for it.

## Longings for paradise, Santa Cruz Mountains, 2011

In the late-2000s, Stephen moved to northern California, caught another wife, left another child. Only Peter now remained in LA, composing and producing music for the entertainment industry.

I drove Highway 17 from Silicon Valley to Scotts Valley in the mountains above the Pacific Ocean to visit Stephen. We talked on his porch, his skin blotchy, jaw hollowed. Life and alcohol turned my invulnerable older brother into a stretched, toothless old man. Snapped a picture. We didn't call them selfies back then.

When I picked him up for breakfast the next morning, the fresh tequila bottle from the night before now stood on his coffee table half empty. I drove us through ancient redwood forests and grasslands with pumas. We paused at a lovely picnic spot; I took a deep breath of the mountains, sea air, and evergreen. Pacific fog patches surrounded two city boys, stretching our legs, lingering at the picnic tables. "What made you quit LA? Your new lady?"

"Are you kidding?" he scoffed. "That got me here." He waves at the surroundings — green mountains, roads winding in and out of the morning fog.

"Paradise." Then, "hey, what was that game your girls wanted? I should have bought it for them."

"That was a long time ago, Stephen. Game Boy."

"That would've shown Dad. I should have bought them Game Boys."

He brought up the girls, then made it about Dad. Stuck in bygone patterns. "They were kids. What they wish for now is for you to become healthy. Erica will have her own baby soon. You're gonna be the extra cool uncle. Uncle Steve."

He stepped back, eyes tightened. Maybe he really wanted to talk about his own children and couldn't. We stood in the fog, the tree's green curtain poking through. "All I wanted was to succeed. Now I know, the people who make it are born there or get lucky."

Say it, dammit, open your mouth and tell him: Stephen, you're better than basing your life on others' terms. You're my brother, not a cautionary tale, the person who understands what we went through. You don't care what others think.

To make it? You measure your worth against shifting external values. And then end up here, in this beautiful place, sick, friendless, addicted, practically an invalid.

What about your kids, in California, in Florida. What would happen to them? But I lacked the guts to ask. Tell him about the Buddhist concept of impermanence. By basing our happiness on stuff that is bound to fade, our happiness will also evaporate.

But I didn't. My mouth wouldn't move.

Scrambling, seeking an entry point, "What about hard work, the American dream? All that?"

He scrutinized me, squinting, as if I sounded sarcastic. "I worked hard; made the Ferrari pit team. You always judged me, Keith."


We went to an AA meeting together in Santa Cruz and I drove him on errands — a drugstore, an impound lot. His car had been seized and licence revoked. It was all a misunderstanding or someone did him wrong or some story. Fortunately, Stephen wasn't one for stories, and I didn't care. I visited to lend a hand and to be together. We'd gone decades with only sporadic contact.

After the AA meeting, we took a stroll on the beach. We met an amateur astronomer, with a contraption that allowed him to directly view the sun. Stephen became like a little kid again, couldn't stand still, and connected with the guy. Within seconds, they talked about astronomy and gadgets and the best burger joint in Atlanta, Georgia. Babies, dogs, and strangers — Stephen had the magic. Standing by his side, I became, again, the apprentice.

## Decisions, Calgary

Several months after visiting Stephen, my bowels blocked, shutting down. My other organs failed once the bowels ceased functioning. Inflammation thickened the intestinal wall, narrowing the passage. Scar tissue from old surgeries twisted and adhered to a narrowed section. It took another emergency surgery to save my life. They removed the blocked section and reattached the healthier bits.

A few days after the surgery, I recovered at home, going back and forth to the hospital for after-care. A doctor in California phoned. She said I best hurry to the Dominican Hospital in Santa Cruz. Stephen was very sick. He had little time left. Questions required answering; someone needed to make serious decisions.

"Decisions?"

"Regarding Stephen's care, treatment. We can discuss all this in person."

I called my doctor. I have to go to California; my brother's sick.

Don't lift. Take your temp twice a day for infection. Do you need anything for pain?

Yes, please. Something strong. The good stuff.

Any problem, have the doctors in California phone me. See me when you return.

## Wound management

As I lay on a gurney in a room named Wound Management, a nurse taught Yoshiko how to clean and sterilize me, and how to change my dressing. "You're still recovering from surgery. Recuperation starts in a few weeks."

I didn't grasp the difference, but the nurse kept going, "Don't lift. You can't lift for weeks."

The nurse filled an enormous bag. In went abdominal pads, wound seals, sponges, gloves, bandage rolls, plastic forceps, syringes, single-use antiseptics, goops and liquids. She piled it on. She handed the bag to Yoshiko, then inspected me, "You don't lift."

On the ride home, I received another call. An angry voice belonged to Stephen's landlady. "When are you coming to clear out his stuff?"

"How did you get this number?"

"Stephen left it as his contact."

"You realize I am in Canada. I just had major surgery."

"Just get rid of his stuff by this weekend or I'm seizing it."

Back home, I phoned Dad, filled him in. "Dad, we will have to decide about treatment and care."

"Make sure they take care of him. Call me as soon as you find out how he is. Try to bring him up here."

I phoned a friend in California. "James, do you know where Scotts Valley is? Can you meet me there?"

Yoshiko gathered the supplies from the Wound Management nurse in a carry-on bag. We were not sure how to pass these liquids and things through airport security or US Customs. Into another carry-on goes our change of clothes and two tickets to San Francisco.

## Yoshiko's story, Scotts Valley

I drove Highway 17 to Scotts Valley. Keith sat in the passenger seat on his phone to Ira. Ira's hearing was almost gone, so Keith yelled. The traffic flew and the highway twisted.

I pulled up to Stephen's house. Outside, overgrown jade and rosemary bushes needed pruning. I felt envy. In Calgary I must baby my tiny jade and rosemary plants and keep them indoors for eight months of the year.

James waited for us on the front lawn, relaxing on a lawn chair, chatting with a woman reclining next to him, smoking. That's not James' wife — Anna Belle doesn't smoke. The woman, the landlady, demanded we clear out Stephen's stuff.

Keith left with the car to the hospital in Santa Cruz, while James and I got to work. The landlady followed us into Stephen's room. Years before, we'd visited Stephen in LA. He kept his place neat and organized. He took meticulous care of his clothes, tools, and things.

This room wasn't neat. It might have been a pleasant room once. Against the outside wall, a glass sliding door led to the garden. Curtains and boxes and stuff blocked the soft mountain light. The room reminded me of a college student's dorm, after a party. And a typhoon.

We found the bed dishevelled, filthy. Candy and wrappers littered the floor along with Rolex watches in cases, jewellery boxes, gram scales, some still in new packaging.

I discovered a portable document shredder, brand new. It would cram in my carry-on.

"I'm keeping that," announced the landlady. "I'll tell you what to keep for me."

Cheap candy lay underneath the bed and in the back of drawers. All this in the open and he's hiding candy. We found expensive hardcover cookbooks still in shrink wrap. Apparently, Stephen collected cookbooks like Keith and their mother. Irene had owned dozens going back to the nineteenth century.

Keith phoned from the hospital. The doctors said Stephen wouldn't survive. We needed to clean out his stuff before we left. I told Keith about the watches. Keith didn't care about watches or a case of watches; we'll locate a charity to donate them to. Didn't tell Keith about the cookbooks. Those, he would want, but I'm not carrying heavy cookbooks home.

I discovered old children's books, possibly from Stephen's childhood. And I found small attractive china pieces. Those I will carry home to send to his children. No time to ponder. Empty this room. I'm a moving train. There's no time.

James and I carried his furniture to the backyard. Stephen kept a garden, growing cucumber melons, herbs, and salad vegetables. Irene's green thumb. An old saying goes, "children learn by watching their parents' backs."

We didn't have any boxes, so we made piles in the backyard for rubbish, donations, and stuff his landlady demanded to keep. Lurking, she ordered: "Don't touch nothing in the kitchen. I will keep that."

We rented a truck to carry donations. James called a service to haul stuff to the dump. They came; they checked out our piles and drove away to fetch a larger truck. I requested, "Please bring boxes."

Years earlier, I'd cleaned out Irene's apartment. More of Keith's family secrets stayed with me now. My family. Keith and I felt for every family member: Stephen, his children, and poor Ira, about to lose his precious child.

One pair of beige cargo shorts hung at an awkward angle in his closet. Why hang up shorts? More than hefty, they felt too heavy. Something heavy is in the pocket. James! What is this? Chuckling, James removed a gun from the pocket, took it outside, emptied the bullets into his hand. Smiling, "Welcome to America, Mrs. Robinson. Michael Moore says Canadians have more guns than us."

"Erica's husband is a hunter. I've never held a gun. It's heavy." James phoned the local police to deal with it.

"Find anything else?" He asked.

"Letters from his children. That's not our business. Look at these from Ira and Irene."

I showed James what I'd come across. The envelopes from their mother and father had been carefully opened. The cards or letters left undisturbed, unread. Stephen sliced slits in the envelopes in a way to remove cheques but not read the contents. He went to all that trouble instead of throwing the letters away.

James raised his eyebrows, tilted his head, and chortled again.

The two junk removal guys returned and combed through the pile for the dump. Rummaging through for stuff to resale or repurpose. "Extra charge for mattresses," one said. "County rules."

James negotiated with them, still smiling. Requested their assistance to load the donation truck. Then, the police arrived. James spoke with them. I left them to it, while I kept going like a moving train, still sorting Stephen's life into three piles.

## He was Stephen, Dominican Hospital

The doctor had treated Stephen for over forty hours straight. She came across as caring and professional and haggard, rolling her neck to work out kinks. "I'm Stephen's physician. I phoned you. Stephen's case is complicated." She used words like multi-system distress, comorbidities. He won't survive. The question is how much to intervene along the way? Doctor-words I can't recall. She got the message across.

She took me into the ICU. Rather than a bed, they'd placed him in a trauma chair, with restraints around his legs and torso, tubes and machines. The doctor wanted him upright, rather than prone. Upright would help prevent him from aspirating. I just left an ICU a few days prior, so the routine felt familiar. At least I knew my routine — be engaged, compliant, part of the process, familiar with the system. Compliant, not Stephen.

He was Stephen, but Stephen with yellow-grey, bruised skin. Eyes resisting, his entire body twisted and pulled against the cables, tubes, and restraints. The magician, unable to speak.

"Wa, dee." Talking to me.

"We are chanting for you, bro. Yoshiko is at your place now." His eyes brightened, then turned serious, silent pleading. He'd had multiple strokes, an untold number. Liver and kidney failure. Aspirating.

"Stephen, do you own a birth certificate, a passport?" Even at this late stage, Dad and I kept a fantasy of transporting him to Canada and proper care. Good health-care came as his birth-right. In fact, from all appearances, the Dominican Hospital provided brilliant care.

He made a writing sign, signalling for a pen. Wires connected to his hand like a puppet. I held a piece of paper against the table. He drew a shaky but clear picture showing where to track down his birth certificate. He drew a sketch of a chest of drawers and a card inside a drawer. Wow, pretty cool. Nurse, doctor, check out what Stephen drew; he can't be dying. Look. Magic.

"Well done, big brother, you still have it. I will dig for it back at your house. Anyone else I need to care for? Any other children?"

"Wan, waan. Wan dee." He got through. Wendy. It takes a minute. Not a girl.

A moment ago, the doctor told me his condition was terminal, but look at him, filled with energy, pulling on the cables and restraints. "Sure, Steve. But first you need to swallow without choking yourself. You aspirate. Once you can swallow, we'll clear you out of here. Oh yeah, we are going to Wendy's."

## Business in a locker

The next day, I called on a lawyer, a notary, and the Extra Space Storage office in Santa Cruz. Whatever Stephen's business, he conducted it from a storage locker. It creeped me out, the first, and only, time I'd been inside these places. Locked gates under guard, echoing concrete halls, giant metal cages and boxes held the stuff of lifetimes. Buy stuff to pay money to store stuff. But maybe that is me being my anti-consumerism left-wing judgemental self.

Once we sorted the legal business, Yoshiko, James, and I entered the magician's workshop. Inside a poorly lit locker, we uncovered an entire office set-up for a mail-order or Internet business. The locker held treasures of Stephen's lives. We found antiques from Mom's estate, tens of thousands of dollars worth of tools, mechanic's chests on rollers, and official Ferrari pit coveralls. We also found a hodgepodge of stuff from his hidden lives: shipping supplies, bottles of his urine in stacks, boxes and boxes filled with weird stuff for sale.

We didn't waste time to figure out what he actually did there. His business stayed none of our business. Nobody cares for details; let's just clear this out.

We donated the furniture and tools to a local school's fundraising event. James called the rubbish guys to the locker to haul the rest to the dump.

Back at the hotel, Yoshiko changed my dressings. For three days, we cleaned out his stuff. I met with doctors, hospital administration; phoned Dad. Who the hell was I to make these decisions?

The instructions were to take my temp twice a day, keep me sterile. That proved ambitious; she kept the wound clean. And don't lift. Well, not too much.

We never got to Wendy's.

## I don't see you

I peer in the mirror but my champion is gone. Now that you've left us, I miss your easy strut and the easy way you handled torque wrenches and power equipment. Not missed: you swallowing a half-bottle of tequila before breakfast.

Anyway, I went back to the beach by myself today. No sign of that telescope guy. He wasn't by the boardwalk, the pier, or the surfing museum. You'd made friends with him so easily I half-wondered if he departed with you. A ridiculous thought. You always left alone.

So, I drifted the long beach without you, north along Cliff Drive. My steps dragged, but got all the way to where you and I toured the tidal pools at

Moore Creek and the Natural Bridges. Your footsteps into the tidal pools where land and sea join, neither land nor sea, always land, always sea. I leaned over the pools, peering in, but I couldn't follow you in leaning forward. Your footsteps vanished ahead of me, gone.

The creatures emerged and departed with the tides. The crabs and the sea stars and the snails, and the smaller creatures too, too small to inspect, live entirely between the oozy tides, consuming each other and being born and making slimy microscopic critter love in the wet and the seaweed. Entire living systems exist for hours and then dispersed, gone forever. For them, a few hours held damn near eternity. Observing life in the tidal pools distracted me for a few moments. Still, it would be cool if I could contemplate them one more time with you, Steve.

## Be my little brother, Crematorium

The Pacific fog blanketed the parking lot and grounds outside the Santa Cruz crematorium. A light drizzle rolled down the waiting room windows.

Inside, an attendant asks questions. Excuse me? "Sorry, can you repeat yourself?" I barely heard her. I blinked. My stomach fluttered, then hardened. My mind couldn't grip, so my hand tried. I reached for the bandages underneath my shirt.

Yoshiko plucked my hand away and answered.

The attendant vanished in the fog at the front. Alone, I collapsed on the waiting room sofa. Far away, next to me, Yoshiko dissolved into the sofa. A fog of grief and regret blanketed the room. Everything blurred together: childhood and adulthood, Stephen's magic and abandoned children. He didn't have to be this way. I tried to show him choices. Instead, I drove him further away. We were so different, so alike.

His words came back to me, at me, a jumble of hurt: "You couldn't simply be my little brother. That's all I wanted. I wished for a brother to be with me. You had to fix me. I would have taken care of you. I wanted to take care of you."

In the distance, across the room, the attendant reappeared, her words emerging through the fog: do we have any questions?

"No. Thank you for everything. You've been most comforting."

But Yoshiko, fortunately, has questions around customs, security. The attendant goes over the paper-work with her. Oh, good, they are taking care of everything. Please tend to Stephen. You are going home, big brother, too early.

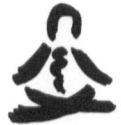

# Coming Home

**A dream of a loom**

I PLACED THE CARTON containing Stephen's remains in my carry-on. Two kilograms of sandy ash and bits of bone. That last night in Santa Cruz, I took pain-killers, something strong, the good stuff. Yoshiko unpacked my belly, cleaned, and wrapped me up again. My carry-on balanced on the side table by our bedside, I slept deeply.

Perhaps opiate induced, I dream of war: bombs flashing, fires. Explosions in the sky. Torching the heavens and ripping and pounding the earth. Desperate for shelter, I dive into a blood soaked muddy trench. I crawl through the mud to the trench's end, which opens into a cave. Statues of Buddhas and Bodhisattvas line the cave, seated on shelves cross-legged. One is different, with blue skin, women's breasts, and one leg uncrossed, pointing down to the cave floor.

Then I am on my belly, wiggling out the cave mouth to hills smoking from the bombs and a vast desert. A caravan, reeking of camel droppings, snakes across the desert. From the cave's exit, rock-strewn hills roll towards the expanse.

On a hill, an old woman at a loom weaves multicoloured sails and ribbon streams. The colours pour out from the loom, into the sky as she works. I approach to determine who she is. She wears glasses and a black abaya with intricate gold embroidery. Her bumpy fingers clasp the shuttle, flying smoothly across the loom's frame.

As I moved closer, the loom resembled a box, like the carton with Stephen's remains. Across the loom's front, I detect writing, but the letters are scrambled, frustrating to read. I must solve the riddle of the words, find the identity of the woman at the loom. The words might read, Steinway & Sons. No, maybe it's Santa Cruz Crematorium. Starts with an 'S.' At her side, rolls of unfinished rugs lie in a stack. At her feet, three children giggle, playing jacks on a finished rug. A gender-less skinny kid minds the three and dances to an antiquated wooden dial radio playing the Rolling Stones, "Shine A Light." The unmistakable playground cadence and children's laughter replaces the radio. The children ignore me, focus on the jacks. I am an observer, watching the children. Not there. If I can understand the children, make them like me, then I will understand who is the weaver.

Back and forth, the weaver's fingers move, like a pianist over a keyboard. Her loom weaves music, replacing the bomb explosions with playful shouts. Red, yellow, and blue form a mandala pattern on the carpet. Her weaving fills the sky, concealing the bomb flashes. Sails and ribbons become flags and woman-made rainbows, coalescing into a mirror pattern of the carpet. The sky becomes a bright warm blanket, bandaging the bomb wounds. A desert expanse stretches past the hills, the same tan colour as Stephen's ashes, scattered with bone and cartilage chunks. The camels and carts passed, but the shit stench lingers. Tracks from the caravan fade into the horizon. Tracks over my brother's ashes and bones. A single cloaked figure with a staff follows the tracks. The tracks go into mountains, a twisty mountain path, alongside Highway 17, cars speeding by, heading home.

We left first thing that morning. With time before our flight, Yoshiko avoided Highway 17 by driving up the coast towards San Francisco. As we passed Half-Moon Bay, I asked her, "Can you smell in a dream?"

## Septic, Calgary, 2011

The day after we returned home with Stephen's ashes, I visited the doctor. It's been less than two weeks since my bowel resection. Checking Yoshiko's work, "You know she's not supposed to do this? No infection signs. Everything is clean. How do you feel?"

"Exhausted. But my stomach seems okay. Tender. I haven't eaten much."

"Bowels moving?"

"Yes."

"You're keeping up your, your . . .?"

"Buddhist practice, oh yes, absolutely."

"Keith, you're really quite lucky. Listen, we need to find another way to manage your disease than surgery. We're getting useful results with immunosuppressants. Once you've recovered, let's talk. Meanwhile, tell Yoshiko her work is flawless. But we'll let Home Care take it from here."

## Rejection

That winter, the doctor put me on a drug designed to prevent transplanted organ rejection. Azathioprine (6-MP) weakens the body's immune response. Since Crohn's behaves like the body rejects its own digestive tract, like organ transplant rejection, they use the drug for both.

The doctors called my reaction to Azathioprine a "one in a million adverse response." Dizzy, faint when standing, a different tiredness, like a tube attached to my head sucked out all my strength. I visited my family doctor. She said I had a cold. Dammit, I recognize a cold. I should have trusted myself. She should have taken my blood pressure.

Within a couple of weeks, I went into shock. Paramedics huddled around my bed, one spoke on his phone, walkie-talkies crackled; they couldn't detect any blood pressure. They inserted a catheter in my neck. PB barked from a shut bathroom. As the EMTs carried me down our stairs and out into the night, a deadly icy blast jolted me alive. This is not the time to fade away. Our minor cul-de-sac filled with blinking lights, a police car, fire engines, and an ambulance. Neighbours directed traffic, far too cold to gawk. Yoshiko wrangled the neighbour's toy terrier.

Before they loaded me, Erica had already climbed in the back of the ambulance. She sat on a padded bench seat next to a paramedic against the ambulance wall. Holding bottles of my meds, she answered questions, going over my history. The ambulance contains a lot of fancy stainless steel equipment. Oxygen tanks and stainless steel cabinets secured against the wall trigger memories. Padded seats hung from the walls, like in a diner. Memories collided. A memory of metal padded seats invades my effort to stay conscious. Fancy medical equipment, tubes with stainless steel caps. A percolator. The oxygen tanks reminded me of an old-fashioned percolator. Shiny chrome. I never asked Stephen what he said to the toddler in the diner, what he did. All these years. You don't ask about magic, you'll ruin the trick, break the spell.

"Wow." I asked the EMT, "What is going on?"

"It's minus fifty," she said.

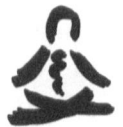

# Gut Feelings

> *The question clearly being asked in an exemplary memoir is "Who am I?" Who, exactly, is this "I" upon whom turns the significance of this story-taken-directly-from-life? On that question, the writer of memoir must deliver. Not with an answer but with depth of inquiry.*[53]
> Vivian Gornick

## ICU thoughts

MY WHO-AM-I STORY BEGAN with questions about blending in. Do my guts belong in my body, or are they destined to be rejected by an immune system gone wrong? Does my life belong in family and community, or am I destined to be "unwanted on voyage?"

Lying in the ICU, recovering from septic shock in 2011, new questions arose. The ICU offered the ideal place to contemplate serious questions. I wanted to join in common cause with a mentor who is of a different generation and background, who speaks a language I do not share. I longed to live up to his absolute faith in each person's dignity and brilliance. I needed to live up to my highest yearnings, be true to the commitment I made as a kid in Sceaux. I could become the person I hoped to be by shifting from craving belonging to creating spaces for belonging, and from imitating authenticity to cultivating value. "Who am I" to be answered through my actions and relationships.

My reaction to the drug did not kill me. I had everything: a teacher and a partner and life. All I need. Except, perhaps, time. Time is in short supply for me, and perhaps, humanity. We must hurry. Lying on the Intensive

Care cot, I would live, no longer searching for the horse called choice. Now, ride.

## Foothills Medical Centre ICU, Winter

My gut doctor came to the ICU, where I recovered from my reaction to the anti-rejection drug. Once he found time, he'd write a paper about my experience and how he almost killed me. "A recognised severe azathioprine side effect is a mimicking of sepsis. But in your case," he said, "no mimicking." He said if I tried the drug again, the chances of going septic again were near nil. No, thanks. I declined.

Next, he spoke about biologics to block the inflammatory response of CD. Biologic TNF blockers successfully treated various autoimmune disorders, he claimed.

With the anti-rejection drugs and biologics, for the first time, we were talking about treatments. This presented me with a new way to relate to my body, my guts, my disease. Since I first got sick as a kid, I ignored my guts, or pretended to. If I couldn't ignore them, I'd hate my guts: they caused my suffering; they held me back from a normal life. Occasionally I'd try to cure them, through gorging, medicine, or supplements.

Carlos had said my broken guts were my gift, my treasure. On good days, I considered how my suffering and experience could be a gift. But my intestines themselves, the physical tube running through me, sure didn't seem like a gift. Honestly, they threatened. I lived with a constant underlying, unadmitted anxiety. How much would my stomach hurt today? What would my intestines deliver tomorrow — abscesses, fistulas, adhesions? How long before their ultimate betrayal? Would a celery string or tangerine segment wrap around scar tissue in a narrowed bowel passage, strangling me inside?

Ignore, hate, fear them. The thing I didn't do, didn't consider, nobody taught me, was to attend to them. As I gradually learned to pay attention to their messages, oh what tales they told. My guts cried out, "Listen to us." I needed to uncover their significance beyond the pain, to tune in to my guts, tap into their instinct and intuition.

As I stumbled through life, figuring out who I was, where I came from, and what to do, my sick guts quietly and thanklessly shaped me. My belly always held a Buddha, offering instinctive wisdom, core identity, strength, courage.

As long as I stayed in my head, denying the messages from my guts, I blocked access to my innate wisdom and made poor choices. Our senses gather information. The head processes sensory input, filtering meaning from noise. Reflecting on the past and planning the future is ideal for the head-brain.

The gut brain processes experience itself, rather than sensory information. Stress, infection, mood, medicines, and what we eat affects our gut microbiome. Our intestines hold all our experiences, a lifetime's experiences, even billions of years of gut evolution.

Cells in the gut lining, called neuropods, secrete chemical messages, hormones, into the bloodstream. I can't think hormones; I can only feel them, if I pay attention. Hormones affect mood, behaviour, emotion, energy. Not thoughts. That is why my gut feelings are feelings, not thoughts. When I chant, I offer all of me — head, heart, guts, my thoughts, emotions, and feelings together — in prayer. In a sense, I become pure vow, intent. I tune in to my gut's intuitive wisdom, an exciting and life enriching endeavour.

The expressions "gut instinct," "gut feel," and "trust your guts" are not merely metaphors. They are biological processes. The gut recognizes danger or safety, reads expressions and body language, and senses sincerity or phoniness. When I pay attention to my gut, I tap my creativity.

As Meghan O'Rourke identified, those with autoimmune diseases might lose their sense of who they are, their core sense of identity. In my case, CD came on early in life with my identity still in development. My sense of self had yet to develop. I didn't enjoy an inner sense of normal. As a result, I scanned the outside for clues to normality. Then, I either mimicked or rejected what I found, often both at the same time.

At the most simple level, our guts provide that core sense of self, who I am and who I am not. Our digestive system winds like a tube through us, from our mouth to our anus. The tube itself is foreign. It has its own evolution and runs semi-autonomously from the rest of us. The guts decide what is us and what is not us, filtering out toxins, while allowing in nutrients. Let's amend the old saying, "you are what you eat" to "you are what you eat that the gut allows."

And courage? The word guts is a synonym for courage. In 2011, researchers at McMaster University worked with a strain of mice characteristically timid. They gave the mice antibiotics, changing their gut microbiome. "Their behavior completely changed," said gastroenterologist Premysl Bercik. "They became bold and adventurous."[54]

The research team tried another experiment. This time they used two mice strains, the timid strain (BALB/c) and a strain known for "courageous, exploratory behavior" (NIH Swiss). The researchers switched the two species' gut microbiome. Nothing else was altered. The bold mice became docile; the docile gained courage.[55]

Human digestive system transplants do not exist. No one is going to offer me a new courageous gut microbiome. I am left with what I have. To find courage and act with courage I must look to my guts as they are. My courage lies in facing reality and discarding fantasy, armed with my ideals and the commitment I made as a teen. Bravery will be in my daily unseen choices to do the right thing, when lots of damn good reasons exist not to.

CD is largely an invisible disease. Looking at me, others noticed not Crohn's fatigue but laziness, not pain stricken but irresponsible, not emotionally stunted but immature. I resisted and resented their judgements while internalising the messages.

Being sick and not appearing sick helped me to consider others afresh. Gradually, my Buddhist practice taught me to turn my focus inward. Taking part in the organisation's initiatives with people from all kinds of backgrounds taught me to look beyond appearances. Perhaps others also suffered behind their smiles.

Listening to my guts required connecting with and paying attention to my body, and then to find connections with others. Researchers uncovered a connection between the gut and wisdom, social connections, and compassion.[56] Sounds crazy, but it's true: the microbial diversity in the intestine affects our loneliness and connections.

My guts are the source of wisdom, courage, creativity, my fullest humanity. There, in my belly, lives a Buddha striving to be set free. Please hear their story:

## The guts sing triumphant

We tell our tale, so you may understand.

Things about us you already realize: Chew, swallow, fart, belch. Shit.
Things you can learn:
How we nourish and keep you safe.

Some you may never learn:
How we sense.
What our amazing world is like.
How we built you.

We wish to raise you, protect you.
Keep you sound.

We are now, only now.
We deliver messages about now.
We hope you listen. Heed us.

We cast messages in many forms
— hormones, peptides, micro-biota, ganglia, neurons,
the vagus nerve. And more.
But it is hard to attract your attention,
when you are in the past or future and we are now.

Who are we?

We are the passageway through you:
Nine metres of teeth, ducts, bags, gates, valves
muscles, microbes, fluids.

This is us:

Mouth
Tongue
Throat
Gullet
Stomach
Entrails
Anus

From our lips to our anus, we weave through you.
We are not you and we are in you;
we put the outside in you.
We were here long before you knew you.

Here before your brain thought.
Before the lungs, we breathed
for three billion years. Before humans crawled,
before feet,
before trees, we were here:
bacteria, viruses, phages, yeast and fungi.
We built the oceans, the sky and now you.

We separate toxins from food.
We remove.
Who belongs,
who is gone.

Your eyes provide sight.
Before there were eyes, we saw.
We get plenty of light,
in our tunnels and pockets and bags,
enough light.

Before there were ears,
we heard the first sounds,
gurgles, streams, soaking gases.

Before your voice
we spoke our thousand species' tongues.
We were here — the first crucible of creation.

We churn; we pound; we mash.

Acids strong enough to melt metal.
Caustic bases to divide, clarify, process.

Cauldrons bake without rage;
we rage without confusion or hate;
our alchemy burns the fires of purification,
stirs digestive sludge.
We turn chaos into brain.
We are joy, dancing without shame.

You fear falling short.
You won't topple.
You can't. We are here.

You cry you are homeless;
we declare your freedom.
You cry you are beaten;
we wind no beaten paths; we are not beaten.
We can not be defeated.
You shall not be defeated.

You cry, you are lonely.
We are many, never alone.
You can not be alone.
We are here. In you.

Before you tell your hands to act,
we clench the fist of liberation;
we guide the fingers of creation.

Use us.
Here we are.

We are thirty trillion strong,
fighting for your single meal.
We are the many, in harmony.

Singing the song before songs,
before voice
We sing the song of evolution, creation, triumph:
Arise!

Feel us singing:
Arise, arise.
Strike.
Shatter the bricks that wall in,
bust the bars that imprison.
You are not done, arise.
We are not dead, we rise.

If you listen we will alert you:
We warn you of the phony, the cheat,
the sly caress of harm.
We foresee the true, the healing,
the warm embrace of care.

We, the impossibly complex,
speak simply, point simply:
This is true; there is the lie,
This is destruction; there is building,
Here lies safety, there approaches danger.

We are now. We cradle chances, choices.
Three thousand choices, now.
Here lies hope;
here is your hope, beyond all despair:
Here find hope.

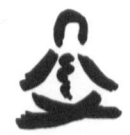

# "Yoshiko, do something. Please."

## Losing my job

ONE OF THE HARDEST periods of my life began ten years ago. 2012 turned into a year of grief. I will tell some of my story. Then Keith will tell of another woman's grief from India long ago.

It started in 2012 after losing Stephen. Keith went septic from the anti-rejection drug. That cold night, he almost died. He hadn't slept in a week. His fingers turned blue and his nails turned purple. He had no blood pressure, and the paramedics said: "Put the dog away and gather Keith's medications. Mrs. Robinson, your husband is in shock and needs a lot of medicine, fast. We need to insert a Central Venous Catheter." Then they cut into his neck.

February first became my last day of work after thirty-two years in the dental business. Five months before, I received a letter from the company lawyer saying my position no longer existed. Then they demoted me and used various ploys to terminate me.

I worked as hard as possible those last five months, staying late every night, after everybody else left for the day.

After I lost my job, I planned to spend more time with PB. Even in the snow and cold, we'd go for walks, enjoy the outdoors. When I visited friends to chant together, PB patiently waited in my car. Afterwards, I'd take him to scamper on Nose Hill.

Those precious moments were gifts PB and I gave each other. He remained healthy, ten years old. I was healthy. This was how we'd be.

Back in 2003, we did not wish to adopt PB. We had no desire for a strong, young, vigorous dog. We grew older and considered slowing down ourselves. But then Keith discovered PB's records with the birth date — September 11, 2001, the day of the terrorist attacks on America. Keith lost a friend on that terrible day and so many people lost so much that day and too many in the wars after. Keith declared, from that day, joy is born; this will be our dog of hope. So we adopted him, and every day for nine years he brought joy to us and friends and strangers.

One morning in late February, we happily walked through thick wet snowflakes, wandering along the frozen Bow River. Wrapped in a white cloud, I said to PB, "Soon I will go to Japan. Let's enjoy today, together."

## Visiting Emiko, March

Days later, I left for Japan to attend a Soka Gakkai conference in Tokyo. After the conference, I met my sister, Chie, who still lives in Tokyo with her husband. We took the train to Yonago City to visit Mom in the nursing home.

We met in the nursing home common room, sitting on a couch with a pleasant outdoor view. Through the large second-floor window, Mom enjoyed viewing a park and mountains. The view reminded her of her childhood home. The chief nurse joined us.

Mom said, "I am ready to go see your father now."

Chie said: "Mom, I am not sure that's a good idea. It's been a long time. Over thirty-five years. This old lady shows up to meet Daddy. He might not recognize you. 'Who is this old lady?'"

After the visit, Chie and I stood in the nursing home's parking lot and Mom stared down from the large window. She stared at me. Her face at the window is locked in my heart. That is how we made our goodbyes.

## Losing PB

Back in Tokyo at Chie's place, they treated me to a wonderful sushi dinner to celebrate my birthday. We enjoyed it so much and then we took a stroll through the neighbourhood with their two Jack Russell terriers. Keith called while we were walking. "I'm so sorry. We lost him."

From a tranquil state, I plummeted to hell. I don't recall how I got back to my sister's house or how I came home to Canada. Losing PB on my birthday is my only memory.

On March 16, we collected his ashes. Emotions choked my heart. Every day, I miss him.

For days after, neighbours and strangers came to the door or left cards in the mailbox. How PB cheered them up, how PB had been their unsociable puppy's only friend.

## Working for Victoria

Soon after that, I received a phone call from my old friend Victoria. She needed aid to take care of her husband. He had been in the hospital with terminal prostate cancer. "I am bringing Oliver home. He will recover at home. If he stays at that hospital, he will die. If I care for him at home, he will live. Yoshiko, help me."

The doctors agreed Oliver would die soon. But Victoria disagreed. If she put all her effort and love and care into tending him, he'd revive. He would stay alive.

But the doctors knew. After three months, he passed away.

At first, I assisted Victoria with house chores. She cared for Oliver and managed the house. Whatever she did, I supported her. At first, I walked her miniature schnauzer, ran errands, and prepared lunch.

Next, I assisted in towel bathing Oliver. After a month, Victoria realized the ad hoc home care nurses and helpers were not enough. She needed the continuous care of a dedicated nurse. She hired a personal nurse with experience in this kind of work, Casandra, a capable and cheerful professional. So Casandra and I worked together amicably.

After a short time, Victoria could no longer take care of the house, so I became more involved with household chores. Casandra and I worked hard. She had a positive attitude and we chuckled trying to raise the household spirit. Casandra understood Oliver would not survive, so we did everything in our power to fill his last days with as much joy as possible.

We moved Oliver to a special hospital bed in the living room next to the patio door. One late spring afternoon, we had a grand lunch. I barbecued steaks and chicken thighs marinated in orange juice, prepared zucchini and potatoes with a raw salad. The barbeque stove stood just outside the patio door. Friends and Casandra and her nursing boss and Oliver's sister and brother-in-law all came. Everybody enjoyed chatting about happier times while I carried food in and out. Oliver asked what's going on, what was all the noise and excitement. He enjoyed the steak, the best Alberta beef, and for a few minutes, he pushed the pain away. In fact, he was in terrible pain.

Oliver was loved. People came every day, relatives and friends, some from far away. I welcomed them and took care of them. People said goodbye in moments of deep sadness. People shared memories in moments of joy and laughter. And people maneuvered for inheritance in dramatic moments. That is how families are.

## Losing Oliver

Oliver's bed in the living room gave a marvellous view of the garden at the back of the house. Outside his window, lilac trees bloomed. The apple tree flowers had fallen, wind rustled the branches of apple trees and evergreen trees. Outside was lovely mid-June weather.

The nurses gave Oliver morphine and more morphine, but nothing relieved his terrible pain. He suffered so much. And Victoria suffered so much, witnessing her strong, vital man in torment. She stared at me with all these people around, her face clouded by confusion and fear, and said, "Yoshiko, do something. Please."

I slid closer to him and said, "Oliver, this is my gift to you." And I sang a Japanese lullaby, the Crow's Song, which I used to sing to our girls. But by then, he needed more than a lullaby.

I asked Victoria, "May I recite the Lotus Sutra?"

"Please, Yoshiko."

So, with six or seven people observing, I recited the Lotus Sutra. And I chanted Nam-myoho-renge-kyo. I continued chanting. While I chanted, Oliver's drugged and pained eyes focused, and his pain softened, and his gaze gripped mine.

"Don't stop Yoshiko, don't stop." So, I kept chanting with everybody staring. I don't recall for how long, but finally, completely exhausted, he shut his eyes and slept.

At 5:30 the next morning, Victoria phoned. "Yoshiko, Oliver passed away. Come now. I want you to come back to the house and do the same ceremony as last night. Please."

So, I grabbed clothes and at 6 am, at their house, I recited the Lotus Sutra again and chanted. Oliver's face seemed softened, not suffering, no longer in anguish.

With Oliver gone, I worried about Victoria. My dear friend of many years came apart. Angry. Sad. Confused. And when the mortuary people came, we took her upstairs so she would not see them put Oliver in a bag. I don't think she remembers, and I don't need to tell. The grief stages don't arrive in stages. They don't come in waves. They don't come on schedules and sometimes they don't arrive at all. But we need to welcome the grief.

## Losing Emiko, August

In the meantime, Mom deteriorated. She was dying too. Mom often said to come see her while she is well enough to recognize me. I spoke to the chief nurse at her nursing home. She said, "Your mother is critical. She doesn't recognize anyone. But if you return, she will recognize you."

Naturally, I was torn. Victoria was a mess. Should I fly to Japan? Should I look after Victoria? I phoned my brother. No answer. I phoned my sister. No answer.

The night she passed away, she showed up in my dream. In my dream, I was at home in Calgary. The doorbell rang. I raced to the front entrance, but of our home in Aino, not Calgary. Mom stood at the entrance to come inside and the nursing home chief nurse stood behind her. But my Mom seemed young, like a young girl with a child's soup bowl haircut. I said, "Mom, you look young now."

So, maybe Chie got it right and Mom didn't wish to show up in death as an old lady. Maybe that's why, at least in my dream, she appeared so young. And very calm.

That morning, I called my brother. No answer. For twenty-four hours, I tried to reach my family. Yusaku was heading home from a business trip. He left a message on Keith's voice-mail, but Keith only understood one word: funeral. "Lost in translation. That can't be right, nobody died. They would have told us if Emiko passed."

"I dreamt about my Mom last night. She looked like a little girl."

"Why'd he call me? Something must be up." Keith said. "Phone your sister's office. They'll tell you where she is."

I phoned her company in Tokyo, surprised when her daughter answered. She was minding the office. "Auntie, grandma passed away. They are conducting the funeral right now, back home. Call them now. Phone my mom." She gave me Chie's cell number.

I phoned Chie, and she said: "We are in the midst of the funeral. Mommy is right here in the casket."

"Can you put your cell phone to mommy's ear?"

She did. I said: "This is my last time to speak with you, Mom. Thank you very much for being my mother. Thank you for bringing me into this beautiful world. I appreciate you so much."

So few words. So much emotion choked my heart.

Before Mom passed away, my brother and his wife took good care of her. Later, he told me about a conversation he had with Mom. Mom told him, "Yo-chan fulfilled our dreams."

I discovered purpose in all I experienced and continue to find meaning in my problems. I am so proud to be Emiko and Tokuzo's daughter. Mommy escaped from Manchuria and lost my brother. But she rebuilt her life, always considering how to help others. Daddy endured three and a half years in forced labour camps without losing his dignity or hope.

He introduced us to Soka Buddhism and showed others how to overcome hardships. Because they survived, I am here today. How proud I am to be a dirt farmer's daughter. I've always had mud on my face and I am proud to have mud on my face.

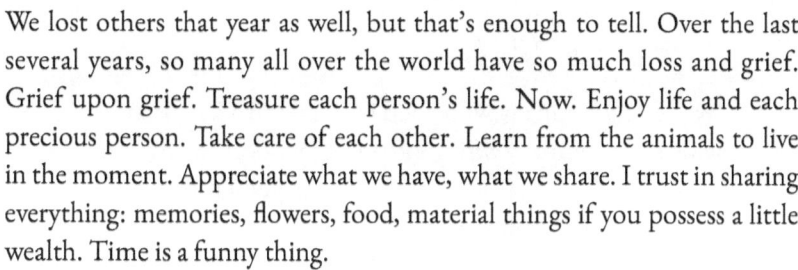

We lost others that year as well, but that's enough to tell. Over the last several years, so many all over the world have so much loss and grief. Grief upon grief. Treasure each person's life. Now. Enjoy life and each precious person. Take care of each other. Learn from the animals to live in the moment. Appreciate what we have, what we share. I trust in sharing everything: memories, flowers, food, material things if you possess a little wealth. Time is a funny thing.

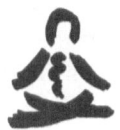

# The Buddha's Friend

By keeping company with good friends even a fool becomes wise. Keep company with good people, wisdom increases for those who do. By keeping company with good people one is freed from every suffering.[57]
Kisa Gotami

## Srāvastī, Kingdom of Kosala 415 BCE

KISA GOTAMI HAD A tough life. Even her name, Kisa, implied skinny, poor, lacking. Skinny Gotami. In those days, to be skinny meant to be despised, a sign of poverty. When she turned twelve, her impoverished family sent her to be married to a merchant in Kosala's capital, Srāvastī. They hoped the merchant would at least put a little food into her.

The merchant cheated customers, mistreated retainers, and kicked stray dogs in the streets. Not a nice man, he mistreated Kisa. He liked to guzzle sura. When he drank, he became abusive. The details are gratuitous. You can imagine.

The merchant's family also despised and belittled her for her poor background. Her own family showed no sympathy. After all, she lived in a wealthy man's house. She had no cause to complain. And they had their own troubles. So, Kisa suffered alone.

The merchant got her pregnant. Her life became somewhat better. The merchant understood he could not beat or starve the woman who carried his child.

Kisa gave birth to a son. Her life became slightly better still. The merchant now had a son, an heir, boffo news for the merchant, and somewhat good news for Kisa.

## Fire and fight

One night, the merchant drank until he passed out. Kisa lay with her son, now two, in the nursery. She patted the boy's head. A few peaceful hours with her darling. Precious moments not to be wasted with sleep. She reflected on how life had become, if not happy, tolerable. The gods granted me a son and my son becomes my lord. I am tied to him, to care for the home and carry out my duties. Nothing can happen in this house without me doin' it. My husband's bliss depends on me. He is now tied to me.

She dozed as the baby slept. For a brief time, Kisa was not alone. Having a son gave her credibility with the merchant, his family, and society. She had become somebody, the mother of the merchant's heir. Society bound a woman's position to a male. Without her son, she was skinny, nothing. Skinny Gotami's eyes popped open in the dark.

A sound woke her. Footsteps, voices. She hurried outside to investigate. In the courtyard, two hands in the dark seized her, knocked her down, ripped her nightwear. She stumbled to her feet. A hand on her shoulder. She twisted to escape. A fist glanced her face. Flames illuminated a bearded, scarred face. Flames. Scars. The man's body pressed against her sinewy frame, a leg between her legs. Strong hands snatched at her tough, skinny body. They pulled at each other, slapping and shoving. She kept twisting, not letting him grip her. As she struggled, her eyes stung with smoke. The fire crackled. Fire in her house.

The baby! She screamed, a sound like a wild animal; flames reflected orange off bared teeth. She punched and kicked and clutched a handful of hair. Her assailant's gasps turned to whelps of pain as she pulled the hair towards her mouth and her teeth sunk into flesh. Hard. He screamed. Blood splattered. Hands knocked her away, her savage grasp released.

Kisa rushed back inside the now blazing house. No sane man would follow her into the flames. As she picked her way through the house, the town bells clanged. A single, terrifying, high-pitched shriek rang out, then choked coughing. She made her way through the intensifying fire. Flames engulfed her marriage bed, but not the nursery, yet. Smoke poured into the nursery. She fell to the floor, crawling below the smoke, and reached the bed. She grabbed the baby and fled back outside, clasping him to her breast.

At Kisa's breast, the baby did not feed or fuss, did not breathe. She put the baby on the ground outside her house and knelt to examine him. No injury or burn signs. His lungs had filled with smoke. He lay still.

Kisa wailed. She clutched the corpse to her breast again, screaming, "Medicine, my baby needs medicine. Somebody, for the gods, fetch medicine."

Bells tolled and the town watchmen cried the alarm. The fire brigade arrived too late to save the house, then turned their efforts to protecting neighbouring buildings. The attackers vanished; they completed their dark duty. Bandits and arsonists, hired by those her husband cheated, had assaulted her and the house. Her husband perished in the flames.

Townspeople gathered at the blaze. Many avoided her. In the light of the glowing embers, others talked to her. "Dear child, your baby is dead. No medicine will save him."

"No, no, no," Kisa cried. "Give me medicine for my sick son. He ain't breathing."

She cried until the morning, wailing through the night. The bells and fire and smoke woke the town. As dawn broke, word spread of the skinny girl prowling the streets in her tattered, soot stained night clothes, calling for medicine.

## Town square

She drifted towards the main square, holding the corpse, calling to empty streets and blank buildings. "Medicine, somebody give my baby medicine. Bring medicine for my son."

Some gathered to gawk at the half-naked, soot-covered, wild-talking, skinny girl. Most people recoiled, calling her crazy. Others spoke in kind tones, "I'm sorry. We can't help you."

She couldn't grasp that her son had died. Loss and a lifetime of isolation and abuse broke her. Kisa Gotami lost her mind, incapable of facing reality, widowed, and barely fifteen years old.

In the morning light, two naked, calloused feet stepped across the dusty square. A thin woman, wearing a brown robe, approached.

"Sister," the woman asked, "What ails you?"

Yasodhara crouched on the ground with Kisa, extending her robe to shield the exposed girl from the gawking eyes. Clutching the corpse, sobbing, Kisa Gotami told Yasodhara everything. How she married a cruel man who perished in the fire the previous night. How she must gain medicine for her sick son.

"My mentor is a skilled physician with powerful medicine. He is at Jeta's Grove, near the city."

Yasodhara stood, whirled towards the staring townspeople, and let loose the full fury of the lioness queen. "People of Srāvastī, are you blind? Behold a great Bodhisattva before you. She has passed through flames to teach you courage, sustained loss to teach compassion, madness to teach wisdom, and endured solitude to teach solidarity."

Kisa cowered, not following Yasodhara's words. Who is this woman, blathering all fancy? What's a Bodhisattva?

Yasodhara continued, calling to the assembled: "Those who clothe and feed a Bodhisattva gather virtue. Those who deny a Bodhisattva clothing will plummet naked into the frozen hells."

People dropped to their knees in shame. Others averted their eyes from the two. A woman handed over a clean sari to cover Kisa's spare frame.

## The colossus

One man, a giant of a man, showed no shame. The colossus lumbered towards the two, reeking of cheap sura and mead and only the gods remember what else. Boozing so early, perhaps he was one of the merchant's enemies, celebrating his demise.

By the hag's robe and shaved head, she must be a witch from the coven at Jeta's. No shave-pated sorcerer's bitch gonna push him around. "Grrrraaa. Nonsense this highfalutin talk of strumpets and saints. I will take the guttersnipe, use her paws in my scullery and her hole in my bed." He towered at least five heads above Yasodhara. "Maybe I'll take both o' yas. Where else you shaved, witch?"

Kisa shrank further, certain she would soon revert to a tormented life.

"Rise, little sister," Yasodhara said, "the lion fears no other beasts and we are his pride."

Kisa stood, trembling. The monster towered above the two diminutive women. His shadow and foul breath enveloped them, the reek of cheap booze erupting from his pores. Surrounding the three, the townspeople rubbernecked.

The older woman proclaimed, "Sir, to slice through the chains of delusion requires a sword much sharper than your few inches of meager meat. Our holes delve as deep as the womb of wisdom. Weigh your words and intentions in the light of the strict law of cause and effect."

The townspeople howled, cheered and jeered at the drunken giant. He hesitated, confused, working through her clever speech.

Yasodhara continued, "Great colossus, your mother carried you for nine moons and suckled you at her breast. She did not thrust you out her hole for you to abuse small girls. You grew to an Asura's size, strapping and stalwart. Use your formidable strength for greater purpose than menacing the weak. Instead, you could be like a demon of yore, sworn to protect the teachers of the wondrous dharma. Your pathetic, putrid twig will become a mighty hardened iron staff, spewing fire."

The giant growled, wavering. A great demon with an iron staff, not bad. There might be somethin' in that. Rumour had it the sorcerer out at Jeta's even hobnobbed with demons.

Then Kisa spoke hesitantly, but she spoke: "You may have me, sir, if you will care for me and my son. If you don't care for us both, I fear you will suffer the same fate as his dear, doomed father."

Kisa's declaration flustered the monster. *The crazy young one offered herself to me. Or was that a curse? Grrraaa, I don't want this mad bony girl and her corpse in my home or anywhere near where I sleep.*

The townspeople roared. "Go back to your cups," one called. "Sleep off your delusions," cried another.

He glanced around, chuckled sheepishly with the others, then slunk off, tromping back to his lair. Thoughts of his mother and demons sobered his tromp. *Yeah, gonna git me an iron staff.*

The townspeople turned their attention to rumours about who set the fire, to speculation about the dead merchant's estate. They gabbled about everything people chatter about when they don't want to acknowledge the suffering before their eyes. They drifted back to the day's errands and annoyances.

## The skilled physician

Yasodhara led Kisa to the public baths. The bathhouse master took a single glance at the odd pair carrying a body. The town bells had disturbed his night and foul talk of arson, murder, and a deranged widow prowling the streets disturbed his morning. He let them enter without charge or question. "Make haste," he instructed them. "When the fire brigades finish their task, they will need the baths. Best they not find two women here, softening the waters."

Kisa clung mindlessly to the corpse, but allowed Yasodhara to bathe her and examine her for wounds. Kisa suffered bruises from the assault and scorching from the fire, but didn't seem seriously injured.

Bathed and clothed, the two marched through the streets. Beneath the remaining smoke wisps, they passed now-open shops, saloons, and artisan studios. Townsfolk stared at the odd convoy: the crazed teen toting a tiny corpse, trailing the fierce elderly woman's resolute strides. The small mad procession trooped out Srāvastī's north gate, over the town moat, and on to the old Sahet Road.

Kisa's eyes remained deranged after the night of assault and fire and death and the morning of terror and humiliation. The older woman's eyes smouldered with a determination that would halt an elephant stampede. She offered to help carry the baby, but Kisa refused, clutching the corpse ever closer. They passed mustard and barley fields, then arrived at the white walnut and mango trees of Jeta's Grove.

Yasodhara did not go inside the Scented Hut. She left Kisa with the attendants outside. The Buddha's attendants attempted to assist Kisa with the corpse, but again she refused to release him. They took her in to meet the Buddha, the World-Honoured One, the skilled physician.

Inside, she found a plain wood and brick space, amply lit by openings in the walls. Simpler than her place, if not for the fire. So, this is the home of the one people talk about. The old woman called him a doctor. The giant said he's a sorcerer. Hope not, I'm already cursed.

Fragrant flowers floated in bowls and incense smoked. His home certainly smelled nice after the hellish stench of her house and her husband burning.

The acolytes gave her a seat on a cushion in front of the dais. An older shaven man in an orange robe sat cross legged, his shoulders and arms wide and beckoning, his torso upright and relaxed. His eyes softly focussed on her. Then, the assistants withdrew to the back.

Kisa knelt on the cushion, still holding the corpse, but no longer clinging to it, holding it out to show the man. She begged the Buddha for medicine.

"Yes, friend." he said. "I will prepare an elixir. But I lack an essential ingredient, a single mustard seed."

None had ever, in her fifteen hard years of abuse and neglect and humiliation, called Kisa friend. The Buddha leaned towards her, reached out his hands and Kisa placed her son's body in his arms.

"A single mustard seed?" She asked. "Sir, ain't hard to fetch a mustard seed around here. Even in the smoking ruins of my home, I can find a mustard seed." The farms around Srāvastī grew mustard. She'd passed mustard fields on their way. Seeds were plentiful.

"Nay, your husband perished there," said the Buddha, cradling the corpse. "The mustard seed must come from a home that has not suffered death."

"But what about here?" asked Kisa Gotami. "Surely this holy place must have a single mustard seed."

"Nay," said the Buddha. "My mother only survived days after my birth. And all whom I've lost number more than the grains of sand along the Ganges River."

"Your mother? I am so sorry, sir." And she was. For the first time since the fire, Kisa felt sadness. A sob escaped her lips.

"Go back to the city, my friend. Locate a home that has not suffered death. Fetch a mustard seed from that home."

## The mustard seed

And so, Kisa Gotami trekked from house to house in the town, carrying the corpse of her dead son, asking for a home where none had perished. In every home she heard stories of those who had died there. Some said, "Everybody dies. That's what happens." Others, "The number who have perished here are uncountable."

The people of the city told of their lost children, lost grandparents, lost lovers. Men collapsed in battle, women lost to floods. Babies to disease. Farmers and untouchables and seamstresses and artisans. Wealthy and destitute. All dead. All born to die. As many as the grains of sand along the Ganges River. Kisa immersed in their stories and told the people her own sad tale. She felt their grief and finally experienced her own grief.

She headed back to the Scented Hut, but first she halted at the charnel house. The keepers followed the Buddha's dharma, so the house accepted all castes, untouchables, and even animals. They gently received the boy's body from Kisa's exhausted arms and reverently wrapped it in linen. The chief attendant said, "In this place cravings end, fear ends. Our bodies, too, are destined here."

## Kisa's awakening

She met the Buddha again. "Lord, I told my story to those in the city, and they told me their stories. We grieved together. In their homes of grief, I found home for my grief. I learned everyone dies, but also gained the benefit of connecting. Through sharing in others grief, I came to grieve the loss of my son and even my husband. All of us, myself and the people I met, are now kin. We are all stronger. That was the medicine you gave me."

And then Kisa Gotami, the woman who passed through fire and ungrievable grief sat with the man who taught a pathway to freedom through suffering. The two friends grieved together. Their tears flowed as one.

Kisa Gotami, the Buddha's friend, became his follower and a central figure in Srāvastī among all those with whom she'd grieved. She never became wealthy. But she became rich, for she enriched the lives of all she'd met. She never became fat, but she became whole. For the rest of her life, she loved and cared for every townsperson, like her own child.

I planted myself in the Philosophical Research Society's library, thirteen years old. I tried to read the story of Kisa Gotami from a 1909 translation. The translation, dry and scholarly, required either some understanding of Pali or more patience than I possessed. Fortunately, recently, I've found a modern, more accessible interpretation of Kisa's words:

When everyone you love is gone
when everything you have
has been taken away,
you'll find the Path
waiting underneath
every rock
on the
road.[58]

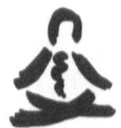

# Friday the 13th

Every six weeks I go to a specialized clinic for an infusion of a biologic medicine, infliximab. By 2015, I'd been on it for three years. The Crohn's entered full remission. My skin cleared and, thanks to the pig implant, the hole in my belly's muscle wall sealed and healed. As long as I made it home for the infusion, we travelled freely, touring the world's wine regions and developing our short-term rental business.

Yoshiko and I visited Paris to attend an Airbnb hosts conference in November 2015. We stayed with our friend Annie and her grown daughter at their apartment in the Porte Dorée quarter on the city's eastern edge. We love Paris' east side — a working class and professional mix, with immigrants from francophone Africa and West Asia. It is not the Paris of high fashion, Chanel No. 5, or tourists. It is the Paris of street art, Tunisian bakeries, and working-class activism.

Friday, November 13th was the conference's next-to-last day. A group of Canadian hosts invited us to a farewell party that evening, but we had one errand first. Sickness kept a musician friend, Brandi, in her apartment for two days. It had to be the worst: a life-time dream of song-writing in Paris, café terraces and inspiration, only to be ill, confined alone in a tiny apartment. Around 6:30 pm, once free from the conference, we took an Uber to her place. The party could wait.

## The Marais, 7:15 PM

From the back of the Uber we people-watched. Crowds along the Canal Saint Martin overflowed into the streets. Wow, lucky people immersed in café culture launching their weekend. We passed the Place de la République filled with Parisians enjoying the fall evening. In the back seat, we shared a smile, observing people celebrating week's end.

The Uber dropped us by the merry-go-round on Rue de Rivoli. At the St. Paul Pharmacy, we told the pharmacist Brandi's symptoms and bought a bunch of medicine. After my usual wrong turns, we located her apartment in the Jewish Quarter.

Our friend is an amazing young woman, the leader of Canada's only all female country and western band, Nice Horse. She runs marathons and is a sailor with the Canadian Forces, a flight attendant, and Airbnb host. A high-energy woman in motion, she visited Paris to write music. But that night, she was sick and laid out. We dropped off the medicine and told her the instructions the pharmacist gave us. Yoshiko gave Brandi the pickled plums she carries for upset stomachs. We talked for a few minutes in her apartment.

"Maybe I will lie down and, if I feel better later, write. Tomorrow, I can jog to the conference."

"You have an impressive attitude." Yoshiko said.

"There is so much we can't control, what happens to us." she said. "The only thing we can control is what we do."

"Hah! You sound like a Buddhist." I said.

We were hungry, tired, and didn't want to lose our way again finding the party. So, we'd skip the party, grab a bite, then head back to Annie's. Two falafel shops stood around the corner from Brandi's flat. One restaurant is famous, named in all the guidebooks. It shut for the Sabbath, Friday evenings. The other, not-as-famous restaurant, stays open on the Sabbath. Customers packed the open shop. Seating inside would be a challenge, so we ordered take-away and stood outside to enjoy our falafel on the crowded street. Yoshiko recognized people from the conference amongst the crowd. They hesitated, intending to dine at the closed restaurant across the narrow street. People appeared crushed: "This was the place the guidebook declared best. Why are they closed on a Friday night?"

Brandi was right. So much of life is uncertain, out of our control. What we do is what matters. Yoshiko reassured them: these falafels were great. For several happy moments, she was a cheerful, unpaid street hawker.

After falafels, we took the Metro to Annie's in the Porte Dorée quarter.

## Porte Dorée

"I held off evening prayers for you. Have you eaten?" Annie asked.

We chanted together until her daughter interrupted. Aurore had messages from friends and social media. North and eastern Paris was erupting with gunfire.

Annie's altar stood next to the floor to ceiling windows and a glass door to the outside veranda. I removed the four of us away from the glass into the salon.

Yoshiko recalls those first moments: "Keith said, let's close the curtains. The fourth-floor apartment overlooked the Porte Dorée intersection. It's normally busy on a Friday evening with a tram station, metro, and exhibition palace. The windows and door to her terrace exposed the apartment and us to the street. As I drew the curtains, I peeked out. The usual crowds and traffic were missing. Duo-toned fire and ambulance sirens wailed 'pin-pon, pin-pon' and the police, 'wee-ooo, wee-ooo.' Police vehicles with lights flashing blocked the streets. Porte Dorée, as I'd never seen before."

Aurore turned on the TV in the salon. Yoshiko sat next to Annie on the couch. Yoshiko and I couldn't follow the French news. Annie and her daughter were catching up, figuring out what was going on, unable to explain anything to us yet. The video showed a stadium being evacuated, interspersed with a graphic of a Paris map studded with red dots. The dots started in the north and spread south and east toward Porte Dorée.

In the salon, I opened France 24 English news on my smartphone, checked CNN International, BBC, then back to France 24. The news was confusing, the situation unclear. What were we facing? What to do? Think. Now.

Yoshiko: "We were in a box, the four of us surrounding the TV in the salon. Outside was unknowable, and the danger lurked inside us, too. Was our box safe? When would this end?"

Take stock. I got up from the salon and moved through the flat, seeing it for the first time. Back to the dining area. The heavy dining table was a potential blockade, where we'd shared *kugelhopf*, Alsatian wine, and joys and troubles. Manoeuvre one of the dining room cabinets to block the door, if it came to that. I inspected one cabinet, overflowing with china and Annie's treasured coffee pot collection, and tested its weight. I racked my brain for ways to lug it across the carpet, into the front hall to block the door, perhaps putting towels underneath to pull it. Well, that idea was nuts. This cabinet was heavy. Tomorrow's headline: "Canadian tourist crushed beneath his own grandiosity."

Within minutes, we received messages and prayers from friends everywhere. "Just tell us you are alive." An automatic Facebook emergency service came into play around then, asking about our location and well-being. The Airbnb conference goers stayed in touch minute-to-minute.

If the power goes out, smartphones and laptops would provide light. I stepped from the dining room to the entrance door hall, checking France 24 on my phone. They reported shootings and bomb explosions at a stadium and elsewhere in the city.

Around half an hour had now passed since the first news broke. I hastened down the hall through the three-bedroom apartment. The window in the far bedroom, our bedroom, offered scant hope if we had to evacuate. I didn't notice a fire escape, so no way out the back, as far as I saw. No way I could scramble out the back window and shimmy down four flights. I'm neither Jason Bourne nor a cat. I snapped up extra chargers, batteries, and plug adaptors from my carry-on in our bedroom.

Keep moving. No, slow down. Think this through.

The cat. If things got nasty, smoke from a bomb or fire, we didn't need to be hunting for the cat. Where was the cat? Back in the salon, on the couch, Annie spoke on her phone, calm, strong, concerned. She didn't glance at me. Aurore positioned herself in front of her PC. Praline purred in Yoshiko's lap.

I plugged in everyone's screens. Allright. Okay. My head felt clear, but thinking somewhat, what's the word, extreme?

Hold on, breathe. Pay attention to me, my body. I needed to pee, and my throat felt parched. I needed water, a lot of water. Breathe. My stomach seethed up and down.

The TV showed live images from the stadium, with ambulances and the field being cleared. Breathe. Deep breath. Heart raced. My phone says 11:04 PM. Now, around an hour since the first messages, and it still wasn't clear what was happening. An hour. Whatever this is, is happening now; not a single incident but something monumental.

A phone rings. They'd turned the TV audio down low, but it reached my ears; I caught only the occasional French word but heard everything. Annie's clear, certain voice on the phone, Praline's purrs, the building's plumbing, sirens distant and near. I heard a lot and understood little. The building elevator's "woosh, ding", the click of doors locking, the building settling. Every sound in the apartment was vivid and distinct, the fridge's hum and Aurore's PC fan, every sound in our refuge. Confusion and clarity together.

Annie's voice was quiet, resolute. I guessed the calls were with her frightened mother, alone in her apartment not far away, Aurore's anxious brother and sister, and with Buddhist friends around the city. Her voice rang clear, a strong, caring foreground over a night of madness. Not the time to interrupt.

I moved into her kitchen, grabbing a glass. Whoa, buddy, careful, you could have broken the glass squeezing it like that. I downed two and a half glasses of tap water. Grabbed three clean glasses and a small tray. Glug, glug, from her Brita pitcher. Glass. Think, did explosions or implosions blast out windows? While the Brita was refilling, I complimented myself for being one of those people who actually refill the Brita. Meanwhile, I hunted Google Translate for duct tape in French.

I carried the tray back to the salon. The TV continued showing live video from around the city, emergency services, and stretchers. Annie, still on the phone, continued speaking quietly, her fine features in total concentration.

At the desk, her daughter texted with both hands flying around her phone, while focussed on the PC, her eyes like two darts. Swaying slightly on the chair, her feet planted wide, Aurore's face had lost its colour. Survival mode. This is my city. It will not sink.

Yoshiko roosted like a mother hen on the floor by the couch; she'd located the cat's brush and groomed Praline. Yoshiko's lips were moving. She might have been chanting. Or comforting Praline.

My hands shook. Annie cleared a space for the tray on the coffee table in the room's centre. The glasses rattled but didn't spill. Annie caught my gaze, her pupils wide. She listened intently on her phone while her glance said thank you. Years before, she had cleared a space in her life and this apartment for us. The flat continued to be, as before, a space of connection, focus not fear, not a bunker under siege.

With Praline under one arm, Yoshiko distributed the water, removed the tray, and tidied the table. Our eyes met and held. Whatever happened, here we were. A Daisen mountain wildflower and me, a boy exploring bushes and bike-paths, seeking a friend, yearning to be a friend. I was so lucky. We were here. We belonged right here. Inside this apartment, inside a world on fire.

Close to midnight, I parked next to Annie on the couch and opened my laptop. The TV showed heavily fortified troops and equipment in front of the Bataclan Concert Hall, four kilometres from us. The national tactical unit arrived at the Bataclan, live on TV. France 24 said terrorists held dozens, possibly hundreds, of hostages inside the Bataclan.

On Facebook, one Canadian from our conference was live-posting the horrors at the Bataclan. A moment of recognition, we'd briefly met at the conference. The woman was in a flat next to the hall. In her flat and on Facebook, posting what she witnessed. What she observed wasn't good.

I glanced at messages people sent her. They read,

> Tell us what you see.
>
> Can you get closer?

Fools. This is real. She's exposed, a sitting duck.

Do something. I froze, my neck bent over my phone and laptop. A chill trembled through me. A sense of dread. Protect us; find safety. Do something. That sick check-mate finality rose in my stomach. It's out there in the real world, it's on TV, on Facebook, nothing I can do. I need to protect and hide. Hide. My hands shook, my fingers rebelling, refusing to press the keys.

People are dying. Tonight. Her, possibly. Stop this. Don't look away. Do not turn away. I managed a series of quick messages:

> Hide. Stop posting.

> Get away from your window, hide as far inside as possible, lie on the floor face down, under a sofa or table. Stop posting.

At 12:20 AM, the military and tactical police launched their rescue mission at the Bataclan. The assault lasted three minutes. They rescued all the hundreds of hostages without injury. Two terrorists died in the rescue. Yoshiko and I fell into bed at two.

## Saturday

The government declared a state of emergency, cancelling our conference and all public events. Aurore left the house at 6 a.m. for her job at a veterinary clinic. Annie would be busy all day. As a Soka leader for much of Paris, she would cancel meetings, while checking on members' safety and encouraging people. That morning, Yoshiko hoped to donate blood. Annie checked with a friend in health care. They said the lines to donate at hospitals stretched for hours and were growing longer. Blood services rarely accept donations from people with Crohn's. Our blood is usually lacking something.

We decided instead to drop in on people we knew who were alone. Nobody should be alone the day after a terrorist attack. We didn't know if it was the day after. The news drew comparisons with the Mumbai attacks of 2008, which extended over several days.

Yoshiko and I visited several friends in eastern Paris and, later in the day, Annie's niece. We passed the Jardin des Plantes. Outside the park gates were planted three flat-black sedans at awkward angles in a no-parking zone. About eight solid guys and a couple of women, athletic-looking and wearing leather jackets, smoked and sipped coffee, faces pale and drawn. The women tied their hair back in ponytails.

No ID hung from their necks; no vests with POLICE stencilled on their backs. They stood like cops everywhere: square posture, backs to the cars or the park fence. No banter. Their bloodshot eyes remained observant while failing to appear nonchalant.

One of the car doors was open. One guy, around our daughters' ages, drooped half-out of the car seat, feet on the sidewalk, talking on his phone. He glanced up from his call, noticed me; with puffy, unwavering eyes. I smiled feebly and saluted, then murmured: "*Vive la France.*"

I wished to thank them and ask if they were ok. But whatever they experienced and did the night before, they weren't ok. But I knew that somehow, one day, they would be.

People cautiously resumed their lives. They were not careless; they were not blasé. On my phone were headlines in English language media, "Fear grips Paris." We observed no grip, no fear. I sent pictures of everyday activities to friends.

Yoshiko: "People were vigilant. They stood up for justice. We understood by their behaviour, a quiet revolution. This force of terror would not defeat them. That's what I sensed from people on the streets, in the metro, in the cafés. In the cafés, they were not merely enjoying themselves. They sent a message: we will win, we will overcome. I really sensed that the next day."

As the day continued, signs materialized in windows, on walls, "We are Paris. Still, we are not afraid. *Même pas peur.*"

## Going home

We returned to Calgary through Amsterdam via KLM, the Netherland's airlines. The Dutch are sturdy folk, renowned for being stoic. What happened surprised me.

Before we boarded at Amsterdam, the crew, ground staff, and passengers observed a minute of silence for the victims of the attacks. On board, our flight attendant, a tall, blonde woman, middle-aged, stood alert, her head upright. Straight out of central casting: capable, professional, calm and calming. She approached me, nobody special, just another fat traveller among hundreds. She asked if we were visiting Calgary.

"No, Calgary is home."

As she leaned in, her face showed lines, an ashen complexion under make-up. Were we visiting Amsterdam?

"No, we've been in Spain and France on wine business. We were in Paris during the attacks."

Questions, one after another. "What did you see? Did you hide? You must have been so scared."

"It was horrible, yes. But we wanted to be with our friends."

She cut me off. "I can't do this." She ran to the back of the plane. I chanted furiously in my head. What to do? Around fifteen minutes later, she came back, but this time pushing a trolley ahead of her. She crouched behind the trolley, her face blocked. I glanced at Yoshiko in the window seat. She must have also been chanting silently. Tears streamed down the flight attendant's face.

Still crouched next to me, she wiped her hands on a towel, squeezed her eyes shut, then reopened them. It came out: today she worked her first flight after November 13th. Before she left home and her three children that morning, her nine-year-old had begged, "Momma please don't go."

What should I say? She bravely wept in front of me. She picked me; looked to me. I would not dismiss either the attacks or her response. But, I didn't know what to say, how not to be cavalier. I said, "it is okay to weep. Everyone is terrified, but we must not live in fear. You are clearly capable, supporting people to relax and transporting us safely home. You must also be a fantastic mother. It is okay to cry. It is not okay to live in fear."

## Blood and Hate

"All the world is aflame," said the Buddha, twenty-five centuries ago. "Burning with the fire of lust, with the fire of hate, with the fire of delusion." Greed. Anger. Ignorance.

I don't know the young men who killed on Friday the thirteenth, for what vengeance or glory they lusted, what they loved or hated, what lies deluded them.

What battle cry sent them to kill and die? They differed, and they were the same as all the young men and women, through time, who heard the summons to blood and hate.

A cell phone rang and young men drove out on a November evening to kill one hundred forty other young people. Because a phone rang or a telegram sent, or a war declared, ships sailed, armies marched. Boys and girls sailed or marched or drove to war for causes that declared justice and occasionally were so, but later, once in their watery graves, meant nothing.

A phone rang, a sermon preached, a king proclaimed words of blood and hate gilded with promises of garlands and glory.

Because of greed: oppression, rejection, machines of control  Because anger: jealousy, wounding  Because ignorance: racism, hatred

Because compassion: the possibility, no matter how faint, of healing  Because love: the possibility of kindredship  Because care: lust, anger, delusion, held and overcome

Because blood and hate: I reduce my isolation through fellowship. Because blood and hate: I join the chorus of community to defeat the calculus of cruelty. Because of blood and hate, I must dance!

# Belonging

And we walked out once more beneath the stars.[59]
Dante Aligheri

## Twist

IN THE AUTUMN OF 2017, Yoshiko and I spent a couple of weeks on a mountain in British Columbia. We minded a ranch with a band of senior horses, chickens, cats, and two immense Australian guardian dogs. As a city boy, I lack experience, skills, or confidence with rural life or livestock.

The dogs protected us, the property, the pets, and livestock from various predators — bears, wolves, coyotes, hawks, and such. The two howled night after night, the amazing sound reverberating off the mountains. Their song penetrated everything with eerie savage glory and kept us from sleeping.

As Lord Byron wrote: "Most glorious night! Thou wert not sent for slumber!" These weren't dogs barking at the moon, but a vibration of raw nature, the voice of night itself. They declared their territory to whatever creatures lurked within earshot. After their day of performing to human order, they employed the night to assert nature's super-rational dominance.

Those nights, we lounged outside on the deck, enjoying the untamed spectacle of thousands of stars.

We enjoyed fall at its best — dripping plums, overripe peaches, rose Russian garlic, and daily eggs. During the day, Yoshiko tended the harvest gardens with gusto, making piles of bruschetta and buckets of tomato sauce.

---

I kept everyone watered and fed and their cages, pens, and stables clean. My duties proved easy, with one exception: the oldest horse, over thirty, needed special attention. Before leaving, the owners told me to segregate old Twist for meals. Twist, toothless, no longer chewed grass. He required his own feed. The others ushered old Twist along when they grazed. My duty was to isolate Twist from the stable twice daily. If fed together with the others, they would bounce him away and tuck into his feed themselves. He'd starve.

The owners didn't share any secrets about how to avoid him or the other horses biting, kicking, or stepping on me. The horses, naturally, knew the routine. Twice a day, as they headed home from grazing and approached me in the stable, they'd clump around Twist. They didn't care if he starved. They treated me like an unruly class treats the substitute teacher. And like an unruly class, they didn't care if they crushed the sub.

The challenge reminded me of river crossing puzzles I did as a kid. My puzzle had one elderly horse, one strong aggressive horse, and seven others. Any of them might kick, chew, or knock me senseless. Hungry living beings, not objects in a puzzle. So, I had to create my own tricks. This required patience, a skill I don't naturally possess. I had to step beyond my comfort zone. I had to hold my horses, as the saying goes.

The only and best help came from Twist himself. At first, I undertook to feed him carrots, hay cubes, and sweet feed by hand. The youngest, largest, and most aggressive horse shoved me away and nipped at Twist's flank.

I read his body language — tightening around his mouth and eyes, trembling legs, his back bowed. The old animal lived in terror — I imagine, of starving, of abuse by his mates, of depending on a stranger. Perhaps he simply deteriorated. As the weakest, he may have sensed the end of his days. I needed to be calm and wasn't. Twice a day, using cues from old Twist, his eye direction, his body language, we'd work together. Using the gates of the corral to direct and a long pole to steer, I separated the one from the others. We danced, the frightened old toothless stallion and the nervous old man.

He taught me. He didn't crush, bite, or kick. For precious moments each day, he led me out of my head.

## Living my own life

That autumn we house-sat through British Columbia, travelling by ferry to the Sunshine Coast. On the ferry in Horseshoe Bay, something happened. One moment felt revelatory.

I stood on the prow. Around the bay, mountains tended to endless generations of the abundant sea and shore and forested coves. Humanity with our troubled selves and troubled communities also passed beneath the gaze of the peaks.

For treasured seconds, my life fully belonged to me. Without shame or doubt or compromise, my body, including my gut, was present. Forty-five years had passed since I met my teacher, since the week I knew would define me. In that sublime moment on the ferry, alone, I reconnected to my commitment to my mentor. From here, all of me goes forward.

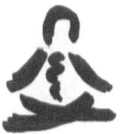

# The Ferry

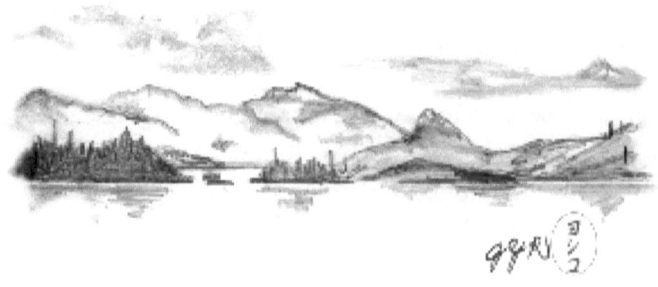

Standing on the bow of the
*Queen of Surrey*,
Inhaling the shifting greys, blues,
and greens of early fall on Horse-
shoe Bay,
Sea, sky, mountains, islands,
and forest arise.
Struck by the scene.

Been treading water
waiting for the epilogue
waiting for the start
waiting for opening night

# THE FERRY

Decades treading water
waiting for the lifting fog
waiting for the rent-to-own
waiting for the cure

Exhausting treading water
waiting for the mystery solved
waiting for the big day
waiting for the muse
someone, someone please press start

Standing on the ferry's bow,
This breath belongs to me.
Not by fluke, not by con, not by deal.
It is mine.
Many hands raised me;
many backs I'd mounted,
many fields tilted in my favour.
But one instant is mine.
This lifetime, mine.

Standing on the ferry's bow,
One breath unclouded.
Perhaps all breaths,
but struck this moment.
Not in spite of my messes
but from choices made
and steps taken.
Oh yes, regrets as well.
I retain them too. Oh, yes.
Utterly unexpected
— this moment on water I belong.

# The Maestro

### "Never be late," February 2018

THE VOICE IN MY head belonged to an early wine mentor: "Don't ever be late for a tasting. Never. It's hard work making wine, and they don't have time to hang around waiting for us. All we do is look cute and sell it. They will be hovering at the vineyard gates, tapping their watches. It is an honour to taste." Brian smiled, teaching. "Don't disgrace yourself by being late."

We were late. Yoshiko settled behind our motionless car's wheel. Hundreds of Barbary sheep stood unmoving on the road in front of the rental car, oblivious to our appointment, or Brian's injunction. Uncertain if this road even went to the Occhipinti winery, I navigated. It rained that morning in Ragusa Province. I phoned ahead to tell them we were late, stuck, and possibly lost. No answer; it's a small winery. Uncertain if I'd reached voicemail, I tried a message — Robinson, Canada, *tardi*.

"Nothing more we can do. At least we are together." That is what we say to each other, whenever lost or in-traffic, or both. Should we reverse through the herd, head back? Surely the flock will drive off the road. They don't graze on asphalt. Find the shepherd, ask if this road takes us to Occhipinti Azienda Agricole. But . . . well, two buts: Google translate, I discovered days prior, doesn't translate to Sicilian, only Italian. And if the shepherd understood Italian, I likely won't follow their response. Anyway, we didn't see a shepherd, human or canine. So, we rested and enjoyed the landscape. "At least we are together."

Mud cloaked the sheep's white coats. Puddles dotted the wet, red sandy soil. The wet ground, covered by Mediterranean scrub, gently rose towards a low mountain ridge. Carob, red oak, wild olive trees punctuated the landscape and low stone walls provided human geometry. We waited at this rough, strangely magnetic intersection of mountain, wet earth, and wet sheep. The rain clouds softened the vibrant Mediterranean light. We sat, unable to go forward or back, uncertain if on the right road. The morning seemed to carry us to this singular place where land and history and sky converge.

## Mother Etna, Sicily

For the previous three weeks we'd driven up and down Mount Etna's slopes, meeting passionate, dedicated winemakers. Europe's largest and most active volcano, Mother Etna, defines their work. Decomposing rivers lava criss-cross their vineyards. Mother Etna's shoulders offer them gifts of moderate climate and adequate rainfall. Under her, they produce unique, unforgettable wines. They create sustainable economic and agriculture models, new ways of living with the earth. Beneath Mother Etna, they proceed gently, respectfully. They don't say, but we guess they fear her anger.

Yoshiko: "Over the years, we've met hundreds of great winemakers all over the world, great farmers, but never like in Sicily. Their dedication and pride run so deep. When tasting their wines, each drop told a story of their honesty and toil and devotion to their place. Meeting them, even briefly, and tasting their sweat and blood became an honour that enriched my life. Each Sicilian winemaker's story made my life fuller, seeing each one's eyes shining with pride in producing from their land. As a poor farmer's daughter, I realize every farmer worries about nature's unpredictability. These wine growers didn't show it, but also dealt with Etna's ash and lava."

Three weeks is not long enough to learn any wine region as complex and ancient as eastern Sicily. But it's long enough to enjoy the best coffee anywhere and devour oranges and pastries made with Bronte pistachios. Yoshiko received her life's best haircut and I, the best shave of mine.

## Meeting Arianna Occhipinti

Today marked our first day out from under Mother Etna's shadow. In Sicily's far south, Vittoria is south of the north African coast, the same latitude as Tunis. In geology also, Vittoria is Africa, not Europe. We thought we drove on a provincial road, Strada Provinciale 68. SP 68 follows an ancient trade route. Twenty-eight centuries ago, Greek colonists hauled wine and oil along it to their port at Kamarina. And probably grazed sheep. SP 68 is also the name of Arianna Occhipinti's flagship wine, whose winery we were to visit.

After ten minutes or so, without whistle, bark, or signal, the entire muddy drove bleated and bore off the road. The road cleared, the clouds cleared, and the sun came out. Yoshiko drove on and found the Occhipinti farm. Nobody loitered at the gate.

An office assistant took us to a tasting room they'd prepared for us. She'd received my message, but didn't understand where we had been, how we got lost? The tasting table seated six in the stone and mortar room, lit by the sun, now streaming through large French doors. A stone forno stood in a corner cloaked in smooth white plaster. A long pizza peel leaned against the oven. Two Burgundy glasses, a water glass, and a side plate lay at each seat at the table. Two bottles of the farm's olive oil and two water carafes centred the thick cherry-wood table.

Our appointment was for a tasting, not a meeting. The owner, the singular Arianna Occhipinti, a poet, philosopher, winemaker, entered the room. She leaned forward in her step, movements precise and firm. Her every move embodied youthful power and ancient culture. I jumped to greet her.

She sat at the table's head, French doors behind, introduced herself, meeting us with steady eye contact, thick black eyebrows raised. Yoshiko sat to her left and then me, my tasting notepad open, pen at hand.

I requested a spittoon from the office lady who brought a basket of palate cleansing bread. Every wine I examine goes through an identical procedure. Not gifted in my senses, I reduce variables in sight, sniff, swirl, smell. With a precise angle of the glass and distance from white paper, I inspect the wine's colour, clarity, viscosity. From different aspects in the glass, I smell each wine four times before tasting. Spit. Write notes. The routine becomes meditative.

Under Arianna's tutelage, we explored her extraordinary creations. Mountains, rock, Mediterranean sky turned liquid through her poetic vision. She describes both herself and her wines as "brave and rebellious." I agree. Her wines embody her life, humanity, culture, and effort.

She explained her philosophy, as if for the first time, quoting Goethe, "'Matter is nothing, what counts is the gesture that made it.'" Not a sales spiel. No sales person quotes Goethe. "I am the first to work with Frappato as the primary grape. Frappato carries grace to power and more . . ." She searched for a word.

"There is a kind of savouriness." I offered.

"Yes, this word 'savoury' . . . it is new to us, but perhaps not new to the glass. It is a good word. I seek balance, not equality, but harmony. You say savoury; I say, bitter and bloody. This land where we grow grapes, the sun rises in layers of red curtains. The road past here is ancient. Once made of stone, narrowing to a single path, now it is the Strada Provinciale 68. Along this road my wines grow, like a discussion, past with future." She speaks with intensity, like poetry. Yet our encounter held a sense of picking up a conversation started before. She tied her long hair back tight. Her thick black eyebrows lifted in confident concentration like inverted crescents. She spoke about biodiversity in the vineyard, biodynamic farming practices.

As she talked, she fingered a corkscrew. We didn't taste while she spoke. Winemakers talk about the soil and what we call *terroir*. Terroir includes geology, climate, soil and subsoil, altitude, aspect to the sun, even culture. These unique elements form a unique grape growing point on the Earth's surface.

All good winemakers realize their wines emerge from terroir, not manufacturing. With Arianna, it is more. Not only her wines, this winemaker and poet-philosopher emerge from the feet of the Hyblaea Mountains, where earth and sky touch. She could not emerge from any other place. Younger than our daughters, Arianna Occhipinti carries purpose in her work. Her purpose puts her together.

Unlike most folk, she showed interest in our experience; where have we been in Vittoria, whom have we met, what terroirs have we tasted?

"We tasted at your uncle's winery earlier this morning. His work with amphorae and biodynamics fascinates me. But they didn't make us late. We became lost, then stuck behind a drove of sheep."

"Why are you interested in Sicilian wines?" She gave me a chance to be pedantic, but I forced myself to keep the story short.

"My primary interest is in wine and spirituality, the vine's relationship to community. To advance from barbarism to civilization," I said, "requires education, mentoring, and rigorous discipline. Years ago, I met a retired genetics professor from the University of Milan. His speciality had been the vine's genetics."

Arianna's entire face widened in recognition. "The maestro!"

I continued, "He told me that western civilization's history and wine's history could not be separated. That much I knew, already. And that Sicily, with its six thousand years of wine culture, formed a microcosm of both."

"Genetics proved this." She finished my thought.

That Milanese professor became her greatest influence, her mentor, her muse, closer than any lover. Her eyes became moist: flashes of molten lava swam in their dark pupils.

Emboldened, I continued, "He told me to begin with Sicily. 'Everything flowed through Sicily, the home, the continent of wine.' Nine years ago, I met Professor Attilio Scienza. Since that day, I prepared to tour Sicily. Now we are here to learn."

Arianna put down her tasting glass, still locking me in her ebony gaze. Her farmer's hand reached across the thick wooden table towards me, fingers dirty from the fields, nails trimmed deeply. "Keith, you and I understand the *maestro a discepolo*, the master and student. We understand each other. We are the . . . the . . . pupils. You will grasp my wines."

# Gardening in the Loire

Until the pandemic, we travelled for Keith's work. In the Spring of 2019, Keith and I worked at a small hotel in the Loire Valley, France. I prepared the gardens for the season and Keith organized the wine cellar, attic, pantry, and storage rooms. We also worked in the restaurant kitchen and turned over the rooms on the regular staff's days off.

It was glorious to gather wild daffodils and to garden in March, impossible in Calgary's climate. I eagerly shopped at the local garden centre for seeds and supplies to brighten up the gardens and planters around the old hotel and grounds. I repurposed chipped tea cups and soup bowls from the pantry as planters for pansies. Using bumblebee yellow paint, I brightened pots to hold geraniums for each patio table.

On the main street in front of the hotel stood neglected planters of lavender, tulips, and daffodils. I cleaned them, adding geraniums and multi-coloured anemones. Every morning, villagers and I exchanged *bonjour* as they passed on their way to the bakery for their morning baguette and cigarettes. And every evening, the same villagers and I traded *bonne soirée* as they fetched their evening baguette and a bouquet of flowers.

Five migrant teenage boys stayed at the hotel. The boys were not refugees or immigrants; they had no legal status. Since they were minors, the French State paid for their room and board. They came from different countries in Africa. They lived together amicably in two rooms of the hotel, kept their rooms neat and took good care of themselves. Separated from their families, in an isolated French village, they shared a corner of the hotel. They spent their days playing footie and phoning their mothers on WhatsApp. On Fridays, they hiked to the mosque in the nearby town.

They reminded me of when I was fifteen, leaving home to attend high school. During the winter, I couldn't go to high school from Aino Village because of the thick snow and poor bus connections back then. An elderly woman and I shared a bathless room in Yonago. On the weekends, I worked at an inn on Daisen mountain. In the summer, I caddied at a golf club. I proudly supported myself, without being a burden to Mom and Dad. Mom and Dad bought my school uniform. Otherwise, I paid for the monthly school fees, food, transportation, and my weekly trip to the public baths. Of course, I was homesick, and that experience helped form my character. Seeing those boys, I am sure they also suffered from homesickness.

They impressed me by how well they took care of their rooms and themselves, and how polite they behaved to everybody. That's why I don't want their lives to be washed away.

The only time they were not polite was arguing with Chef about the food. Like me, they had trouble with the traditional French cuisine. Chef knew not to cook them pork. Otherwise we had day after day of ox-tail terrines, lamb kidneys, and poached veal face. Keith loved every bite. Daddy would have loved it, too. I gagged even thinking about putting it in my mouth. I survived on fresh vegetables, *croissants,* baguettes, and goat cheeses. Day after day, the boys pleaded with Chef for fruit and to cook rice for them. Chef's answer: *"C'est la France."* When they left the kitchen for their rooms, they loaded their arms with fruit.

With unspoken and spoken prejudice, the village people made it clear they weren't welcome. The owner of the house next to the hotel complained about "the monkeys falling out of trees here." The local schools refused to accept them.

I understood prejudice as a child, coming from a poor family and a poor village. My schoolmates, even teachers, ridiculed me.

Until they become adults, the boys would live in the hotel and have to cooperate with the hotel owner and staff. These boys deserved respect. As a mother, I hoped to help them in some way. They told me they hoped to become apprentices or enroll in a technical training program. They called me *maman canada*, and Keith, *poppa boudha*.

What would happen to them, once they were no longer children? They faced a dangerous, unknowable future. But one thing was knowable: their future would be a hundred times harder than anything I experienced.

Behind the hotel near some pomegranate shrubs, the boys strung a laundry line. One sunny afternoon, I hung Keith's and my laundry. One boy folded a pile of shorts, sweatpants, and jerseys. He wore the usual t-shirt and jeans teen uniform. The clothes didn't quite fit, maybe because they were second hand or maybe it's the style? Adeep looked like every other teen, without piercings, tattoos, jewellery, or watch. A normal teen with worries behind cocky teen eyes. Instead of sneakers, today he wore flip-flops. I hung our laundry while Adeep took down his. As Spring went on, the weather warmed, and the pomegranate flowers reddened, and I looked forward to hanging laundry.

---

Ever since, I have thought about them and hoped a small business would take them as apprentices or some school accepts them. I'm afraid they'll end up on the streets of Marseilles or Paris selling tourist trinkets or in the drug trade. A future fleeing the police and authorities is no future. That's not life.

Whenever we returned to France, as a mother and grandmother, I kept an eye out for them and often wondered about them. As a Buddhist, I appreciate our connection and wish for them to fulfill their life's purpose. Their families probably sacrificed everything to send them to France and seek a brighter future. I hope they discover a place they belong in France, contribute to the society that has taken them in, and open the future for their families as well.

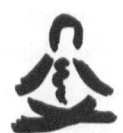

# Blue Buddhas Make Me Whole

## The biologic

SINCE 2012, THE YEAR after Stephen died and after I almost died from the anti-rejection drug, I've been on a biologic medicine, infliximab. Infliximab reduces inflammation by blocking TNF-alpha, part of the body's immune reaction. Infliximab treats other immune system disorders, including rheumatoid arthritis and ankylosing spondylitis. A biologic medicine is a genetically engineered protein fermented from living mouse cells. The process doesn't harm the mice. It is fancy stuff, indeed. For me, and many others, infliximab works.

Fermenting mice cells is complicated. As you might imagine, infliximab is frighteningly expensive. In the fifty years since my doctor told me nothing could be done, other successful treatments have also been developed. If you, dear reader, or one you love, has Crohn's, my point is not to recommend infliximab, nor to claim its efficacy. Each patient has to manage this disease together with their health care team. I do not write this as one of those ubiquitous disclaimers: "seek professional advice." I write this as my experience and heartfelt advice.

Infliximab is not a cure for Crohn's. It shuts down our immune response, so our bodies stop trying to kick out our digestive system. Reduced immune response makes us more susceptible to other issues, of course. Plenty of people will tell you about this or that "cure" for CD. Since, at the time of this writing, no cure exists, I will not be one of those people.

## Short gut

By 2020, I'd been on infliximab for nearly eight years. Other than irregular bowel movements and short-gut syndrome I enjoyed robust health. The Crohn's remained in remission. My skin cleared. The pig collagen biomesh held my innards where they belonged, inside and not protruding through a gaping hernia.

Short-gut syndrome is exactly what it sounds like: surgeries removed much of my large and small bowel. The missing parts absorbed certain vitamins, minerals, protein, fat, calories and other nutrients. The surviving gut tries to make up for what's missing leaving me not anemic, but malnourished.

Short-gut also causes diarrhea and liquid stools, since my gut doesn't absorb all the water it should. It's a mystery exactly how much of me is gone and what remains, but surgeries removed or creatively rearranged various gut structures. I tire easily, probably because of not fully absorbing nutrients. But I am no longer overwhelmed by non-stop Crohn's fatigue. I no longer require two-hour afternoon naps just to function. By any standard, these difficulties are trivial compared to the active CD nightmare that was my life.

## Spain, Roda de Berà, Tarragona, 2020

Our timing could not have been worse. The day before the WHO declared the pandemic, Yoshiko and I flew to Spain for wine business and a rendezvous with an Australian friend. In early March, 2020, coronavirus hit Spain the hardest. Our daughter, Andrea, left for London days before and planned to join us. Oy.

As we landed in Barcelona, our phones crammed with messages cancelling all our travel and business plans and meetings. From the airport, we drove directly into lockdown in Roda de Berà, a Tarragon village. The village was silent, everything shut or shuttering. Needing supplies, but unaware for how long, we faced half empty shelves at the Mercadona Supermarket. In the checkout we inadvertently lined-up too close to the woman just ahead. She swivelled and snarled in our direction, *"dar marcha atrás."* Then in English, "Back off."

The next day Andrea messaged from London, "Trudeau says come home."

How? WestJet booked us on a flight from Paris for March 20. Three days to reach Paris. I located a flight on Veuling, booked and paid for two seats.

By that time, the authorities cancelled all buses, trains, planes, even boats out of Spain. Hours after I paid, they cancelled the Veuling flight and all flights.

We kept our rental car to drive one way to the Paris airport. But, what would happen at the border, would they allow us into France? Nobody knew. The Canadian consulates in Madrid and Paris didn't answer my emails. I contacted a friend who works for the French foreign ministry. Even he didn't know.

———

Yoshiko drove; I navigated, sent texts, emails for work, and browsed the Internet for hints of what would happen when we got to the French border. Leaving might be the wrong choice. Maybe we should stay in the village, hunker down, sit this out. This probably won't last more than a few months. No good, I must be home for my six-week infusion.

The lockdown across Spain shut everything, including most gas stations. We drove through shutdown villages and towns — stores, monuments, schools, all closed. Our car sped alone on the empty thousand kilometre four lane Autopista del Mediterráneo.

I expected sirens, soldiers by the truckloads rushing to enforce the lockdown. Instead, we drove inside silence and emptiness. We drove through a Barcelona devoid of traffic and beneath the teeth of the mountains of Montserrat. Our car hurtled north alone, but we were not alone. Those early pandemic days, the world drove blind.

## Franco Spanish border

The Internet said anyone outside of their homes in France had to have a document declaring a stipulated, legitimate purpose. The stipulated purposes didn't include going home from Spain to Canada. Without the form or ability to print one, I improvised my own on a blank sheet of paper in my horrible French and even more horrible handwriting.

That afternoon, we crossed the Pyrenees Mountains and drove down into France. Along the freeway, hundreds of stopped semi-trailers lined back up the mountains for miles. Passing the line-up we arrived at the French side where a couple of police cars sat. No other passenger cars. No clipboards, hazmat suits, or vans from the Health Ministry.

Barricades blocked the freeway's opposite side, the going back-to-Spain side. For the first time since 1995, the authorities sealed the French-Spanish frontier. Once in France we had no way back.

A cop waved us over. I pulled out everything — passport, driver's license, International Driver's License (only three years expired), rental car agreement, boarding passes on my phone. I leaned across Yoshiko from the passenger seat brandishing my handwritten declaration. With no justification, I felt proud of my document. My homemade, illegible paper should grant us uninhibited passage.

The masked cop kept his distance, asking us questions we didn't understand. Masked, I attempted to answer. More masked cops gathered around the car, meaning well, while keeping distant. The cops and I all talked, muffled, incomprehensible to one another, like humans and dolphins through aquarium glass.

More cops congregated, speaking on cell phones, two-way radios on their belts squawking. Our car became an island surrounded by yakking, helpful cops. A masked charades game, with all the players trying to be supportive, trying to be understood, and trying to keep their distance.

Me, I waved documents at the cops with one hand while my other hand pressed my handmade document against the window.

An unmasked cop confidently strode across the freeway towards us. The cluster around our car parted. His confident bearing and handsome cognac-brown face exuded good energy. His eyes said, let's solve a problem. He and Yoshiko would put an end to my silly, earnest dance.

He ignored me and the papers I waved. His leather gloved hand rested comfortably on the driver's door. "Madame, where are you going?"

"Charles de Gaulle Airport."

"And this car, where is it from?"

"It's a rental."

"Ah," the other cops nodded, "*D'accord. l'Aeroport.*"

After a cursory (and, I imagined, disdainful) glance at me, "Madame, please have a safe journey."

And she drove us into France.

## Le Grand Hôtel Molière, Pezenas, France

That night we stayed at the Grand Hôtel Molière, southern France, with no staff and no other guests. How grand indeed, having the entire nineteenth century hotel to ourselves. Our accommodations came complete with a grand piano and bust of the playwright and satirist Molière in the lobby. Lockdown closed everything in town; all stores and restaurants had shut.

I sterilized every surface in the hotel room, losing track of how many times I touched my face. Fortunately, Yoshiko had prepared the fridge contents back in Tarragona. Yoshiko spread a grand picnic of potatoes and carrots, boiled eggs, crackers, Spanish bread, sweet pepper and fennel slices, Valencia oranges, goat and sheep cheeses.

We'd made it to France; Andrea caught her flight from London home. Gratitude makes every bite tastier, and this dinner in an abandoned hotel became a feast. The two of us relished a memorable meal in our private sanctuary. We chatted quietly, aware that everyone outside our empty stone hotel faced the same certainty that uncertainty lay ahead.

Back on the road, early the second morning, I dozed as Yoshiko drove. A slight jostle at a bridge joint woke me. My eyes opened to the world's highest cabled bridge, the Millau Viaduct. Ahead floated a series of woven steel threads. Three hundred forty three metres below us were the towers, gorges and fields of the thirteenth century Kingdom of Aragon. No other cars or trucks in any direction. With cable stays shaped like sails, light clouds floating below, we briefly floated high above the gathering troubles of 2020.

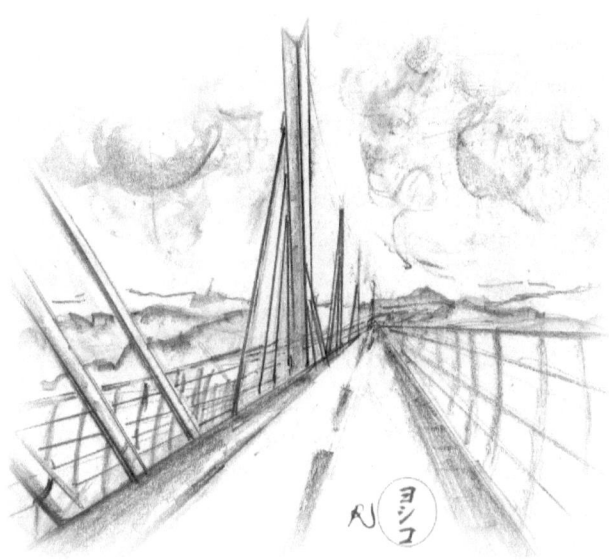

## Kidneys fail

We came home on WestJet's second to last flight out. Our four small businesses quickly shut down, but we were home and safe and contented. I stayed home and baked bread. Many did not stay home and bake bread. Many had to work, often at risk to themselves and their families. Others, in prisons, long-term care centres, and hospitals, died. At the time I write this in November, 2022, some 6.6 million have died, never to bake or eat bread again.[60]

I could not float above the difficulties. While seeking ways to be useful, I began assembling these stories and memories.

After our obligatory quarantine, I fell ill. My symptoms differed from Crohn's or Covid. Towards July's end, they hospitalized me for kidney failure. They drained over 1600 MLs of urine out of my bladder. They said a normal bladder is full at 500 MLs. My urine backed up into my kidneys, damaging them and threatening to kill me. I stayed at the Foothills Hospital for almost two weeks. They stabilized me, made sure I didn't die.

But they did not say what was wrong.

They sent me home with my kidneys stabilized, symptoms under control, and tubes coming out of places you don't want tubes coming out. While I waited to meet with a specialist, home care nurses came to the house to care for the tubes. I washed and maintained the bags that accompanied me at night and the smaller bags for the day. After several months, a urologist examined me. Young, bright, and caring, he listened to my story attentively. He scoped inside me. I needed surgery.

---

At 6 am, surgery day, October 2, I chanted simultaneously with concerned friends. After Yoshiko woke, we did our morning prayers and chanted together. We had time before heading to the hospital, so we did morning prayers again. Why not? And chanted more.

After we finished chanting, I wrote "Surgery Morning Haiku:"

> Gold leaves in a pile
> The surgeon's knife awaiting
> This instalment ends.

Every time surgeons sliced me open, more of me became more vulnerable, more exposed. The surgeon sees more of me than anyone else; they see my hidden trauma. They cut me to heal me. Cutting, whether to heal or harm, alters me in ways lasting and undefinable. My life is often in others hands — my flight's pilot, the Uber driver, all the other drivers on Highway 17. Unlike the others, the surgeon examines inside me when I am in distress, afraid, and naked.

## The alchemist's studio

At the hospital, I met with the anesthesiologist. He posed the usual anesthesiologist questions around allergies, previous surgeries, and heart condition.

He said, "we can go either of two ways — we can put you out or perform an epidural, a spinal block."

"Let's do an epidural. But I have one condition. Keep me awake. I want to be awake for everything."

"That's not usually how this works. I will try, but the meds are powerful. You might stay awake, but you will probably be out of it."

They took away my glasses, disorienting me. They took me into the operating room. The caring young urologist, completely cloaked, welcomed me. Lots of people in full PPE worked on futuristic high-tech instruments. Every corner of the room held robotic surgical machines and electronic screens and shiny equipment. They rolled me on a gurney into a scene from a science fiction movie. The urologist even wore a strange Borg-esque apparatus over his eyes. Masked and cloaked from tip to toe, the team readied for me.

The anesthesiologist said, "Now you will feel wonky," as Morpheus said to Nero.

I became disoriented; yup, wonky. Here came the scene where aliens abduct the hero and probe him and perform horrific procedures on him. They might remove part of him, or they might implant an extra, alien part in him. Maybe both.

But I determined to be present and stay awake. I said to myself, "My name is Keith Robinson. I am a bodhisattva of the earth. Born in Vancouver, BC. My name is Keith Robinson. I am a bodhisattva of the earth. My name is . . ." Over and over. I stayed alert and present for the entire operation. I interacted properly with the doctors and nurses. They worked hard but took the time to explain everything, answer my questions.

Alien no longer, the surgeon morphed into a grand alchemist, the maestro of his sacred, sterile studio. He peered inside me through a scope viewing device while each hand steered wand-like rods. The operating theatre became a stage at the threshold of possibility. With microscopic accuracy, his tools penetrate my sex.

Meanwhile, the surgical team mutated into a magician's helpers. They poured wave after wave of life-bringing fluids through my reproductive organs. I continued reciting my name to myself, but that me no longer existed. In one hour, they cracked my identity, fracturing me from the inside. The alchemist continued answering my questions, quietly issuing instructions to his assistants.

The alchemist mutated again. He and his assistants became beautiful healing Buddhas. They wheeled me out.

## The blue Buddhas

I have been in more than my share of recovery rooms, but none like this. Several blue nurse-Buddhas rushed machines to my gurney. I hoped these new post-op Buddhas were the ones to reassemble my parts. On the ceiling ran tracks. Enormous bags of fluid, many times larger than IV bags, hung suspended from the tracks. The bags rolled along the tracks towards me. They pumped the fluid through me.

One nurse, clearly the Buddha-leader, strode confidently in her blue PPE, directing the recovery with precise care. Using tongs, she grasped a glove shaped implement loaded with super-cooled fluid. She placed the glove on different parts of my body, speaking gently. Nothing. I saw the glove touch skin, but sensed nothing. Her other hand held a telephone.

"You're doing great. Do you wish to make a phone call, Mr Robinson?"

You bet I did. I longed to phone the world, tell everybody: in a basement operating room, aliens reconstruct the broken, making us whole again.

## A hidden jewel

Some questions can best be answered in story. Big questions. What is enlightenment? Does life have meaning? Who am I? The Lotus Sutra uses parables to help us find our answers. The Buddha relates some parables. Disciples tell their own parables in response. Back and forth, they form a kind of dialogue rich in metaphor and story.

One parable, "The Jewel in the Robe,"[61] tells of a poor man who visits his wealthy friend. They wined and dined and the poor man dozed off. The wealthy man had to leave on business but yearned to aid his impoverished friend. He sewed a priceless jewel inside his sleeping friend's robe.

The poor man awoke and continued his destitute life, ignorant of the treasure he carried. His life descended from bad to worse, spiralling downward in degenerate failure and despair of the slightest hope. Eventually, they encountered each other again. The wealthy man, shocked by his friend's decline, inquired, "Why didn't you use the jewel to elevate yourself out of poverty?"

"Jewel?" the poor man replied.

The wealthy man showed him the treasure still hidden in the robe. The poor man was overwhelmed by joy. He had the treasure all along, and now he recognized it.

A precious jewel radiates from the glittering centre of us all, reflecting our energy for transformation. It is humanity's birthright.

This ancient parable considers a modern problem — identity and alienation. The poor man suffered from ignorance about his identity, the bearer of a great treasure. We are the poor man, ignorant of our highest selves, our jewel within. We don't recognize our own treasures of generosity, sincerity, courage. Our ignorance impoverishes our bodies, our families, our nations.

The poor man lacked self-respect. He suffered spiritual impoverishment, a scarcity of hope. He didn't recognize his worth. The poor man is me. His story mirrors mine — his descent into ever-deeper poverty mirrors my descent from invisible illness to denied self. At the bottom is confusion over who I am, where I belong. Is my body safe here? Am I safe with my body rebelling against my guts, against itself? What am I worth if I don't even possess my own body?

A couple of weeks after the surgery, I read Nichiren's lecture on the line from the parable, "When the poor man saw the jewel his heart was filled with great joy." Nichiren explains: "This passage refers to the great joy that one experiences understanding for the first time that one's mind from the very beginning has been the Buddha."[62] The jewel is our mind of faith, faith in our own and others' inherent nobility. The poor man isn't poor at all. His identity is resilient, brave, kind.

I put down the book containing Nichiren's thirteenth century lectures. Aliens and alchemists and Buddhas: What did that all mean? I am intact. My kidneys worked again; the tubes, removed. My boy-bits functioned.

I reread the parable. The passage, "his heart was filled with great joy," struck me, as if talking about me. Joyous energy opened my chest and out my shoulders. Joy buzzed through me. I am alive. I leapt up from my seat beaming. I'd won the best lottery.

The next morning, I still wore a silly grin. I am alive; I must take action. The grin stayed with me all day. My journal entry for that day: "A new life begins."

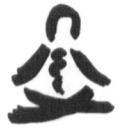

# New Year's Morning, 2021

I went out this morning
Not waiting or anticipating or expecting

With purpose diligently learned in apprenticeship.
To create a passion wrapped gift,
Received from and offered to the noble child,
Teach the silent to be noisy.
Teach the noisy quiet dignity.
Dozens of dark eyed juncos alight as I pass their barren hedge.
Sincere as an elemental ode,
sincere as a horse in a new year's field.

All things will change today:
The outcast, the wretched, the miserables be ennobled,
The fermented rot provides sustenance,
The lovely dark-eyed prostitute and the petty bow-legged thief give lessons on forgiveness,
The horse snorts and pisses on the frozen lump.
And the poet might learn to sweep.

I am here today — awake alive aware
The cold of the air,
my hot breath,
a retriever bounds golden through the snow.
The thief asked,
"where you from, boy, where are you from?"
I answered, "from Kerrisdale."
The horse said, "then get on back."

I feel my body,
No waiting, no anticipation, no expectation
The body is ever in the moment — what's the issue?
I feel my body inside crawling, streaming, and steaming
The stretch of muscles and fascia
around living bone and organs
Generosity from, salutations to, the noble sun.

Among the silent, needless of requital;
among the noisy, needless of validation,
Inspiration from the dark eyed juncos,
inspiration from their leafless home,
Finding joy this day,
Without waiting or anticipation or expectation
This day, my nirvana-joy, containing all days of life and death.

# The Hill

## A search for a connector

ONE BRIGHT WINTER AFTERNOON, I wrote at my desk, searching for a connection that binds these stories I've shared here. Well, here I am, in 2022, in a world on fire, seeking a thread to reconnect our torn hearts and torn world. What connects my story with yours? What links my stomach on fire with our world on fire? In a sense, immune system disorders occur when the body doesn't recognize its connection to certain parts of itself and rejects them.

That afternoon, like many afternoons, the world seemed in the grip of a delusion, going slightly mad. Parts of humanity launch wars against other parts. We poison the water we share and depend on. We go about our lives, deluded, thinking we are alone, separate from the Earth and all its creatures.

There's an urgency in my questions: a sense my clock is ticking down and possibly humanity's as well. I tie my fate to yours, gentle reader, and to our collective fate. Healing our broken world is just as impossible and just as attainable as healing my broken life.

Dazed, disconnected, rejecting parts of ourselves, is it any wonder we hurt, we feel so damn incomplete?

---

The low winter sun shimmered through the study window, first warming my forehead, then striking my eyes. The glare blinded my view of the computer monitor. Draw the curtain, or I could head outside, check for good words in the real world, not on a screen. I pulled on boots with crampons, grabbed a coat and hiking sticks, and headed out, leaving the smartphone, but taking my questions.

## No days off

Swinging the hiking sticks I meandered up the ice patched path, up the steep, frozen hill behind our house. Crystals in the air sprinkled my face. The crampons crunched ice under the light dusting of snow. Shrivelled fruit remained hanging from wild apple trees. Crimson dots from the fallen apples, wild asparagus berries, and creeping wintergreen fruit freckled the pale brown hill. A couple of dogs ran free, in the moment, joyously. A tall athletic guy worked the hill like stadium stairs, jogging up, striding down. He ran past a lone dog, a retriever burrowing through the ice on a berm, ferociously ferreting for mice. As the berm crossed a bushy area, several magpies stockpiled twigs for nests. Not many people on the hill today, leaving me alone with my questions. The temperature stayed tolerable, refreshing, actually.

Further up, I passed through a thicket of leafless Quaking Aspen and poplars. Nichiren's seven hundred year old encouragement came to mind. We are as if in winter, he wrote, but winter always turns to spring.[63] This deep winter day contained the sleeping cause for spring. Woodpeckers typed away at their wooden keyboards, a syncopated tappity-tap. Dead branches offer the perfect over-winter environment for insect colonies. Higher still, I find a single stunted evergreen decorated with red balls, plastic snowflakes and silver tinsel. Someone chose to share holiday cheer with everyone on the hill. Bravo.

Crunch, crunch. My path intersected a man and woman heading downhill. Foothills Medical Centre ID hung from their necks. We chatted, mostly the woman and I, for a minute. She inquired about the crampons attached to my boots, the poles in my hands.

"Safety first. At my age, I can't slip. End up as your customer."

"That's orthopedics. We're in pulmonary care."

"Covid? Is it over?"

"Yeah, the Covid team. No, this isn't over, not yet."

"You must be exhausted. We appreciate all you do. You are the real story, not the headlines. I hope it isn't discouraging. I can't imagine what you've gone through."

The woman replied: "This is what we trained for. Every day we improve. We are learning how to beat it every day."

Then the man. Was it the tone of my voice, or relief at the end of another long shift? Not on duty, his scrubs off, a moment released from his professional role.

"Ah." a soft sigh escaped. "We've lost so many. Patients, colleagues. No days off. No quitting now."

His voice didn't crack, confiding in a stranger. But I heard the grief, and his daily strength working through it.

I wished them well, and at once regretted not saying more. We spoke for only moments, then I continued going up and they continued down.

## What can I do?

Even in the dead of a Calgary winter, the tips of the poplars and lilacs turned dark green, fattening to bud. At the top, a raven cawed.

I spent a couple of minutes at the top, my gaze chasing the raven, then headed back down. Halfway down the hill past a stand of mountain ash, the space opened to an expansive view of the city below. A local resident had cleared a spot, levelled the ground, and constructed a homemade bench of rough lumber. It wasn't a city bench, clearly not the official issue. An anonymous person decided what needed done and did it. Our broken world offers so much reason to despair, yet they took action. Everyone gains.

In summer, the bench provides a welcome rest stop in my meanderings. Catch my breath, enjoy the view, think about life, think about nothing. Inspired by whoever set up this bench, I pick up the occasional cigarette butt or Coke can left on the hill by others.

Winters are usually too cold to sit, but not today. With my glove, I wiped the seat of the thin layer of snow and leaned the hiking poles against the arm of the bench. Comfortable and attentive, I perched. The afternoon light warmed burnt orange, reflecting the orange berries hanging off the ash branches. The sky, now a faded blue, mirrored the juniper berries on the ground around the bench. Took a deep breath. Without thinking, I slid over, taking space and making room.

I should have said more to the doctors on the hill to appreciate their efforts day after day. And my own doctors. For all the shortcomings of modern medicine, they kept me alive.

The Buddha was called the Great Physician. He offered practical therapy, treatment for spiritual and psychological and physical ills. He cured no one. Good medicine does not cure disease. Rather, it activates the body's natural healing ability. Likewise, no single person will cure the problems of humanity. We need to pitch in, trigger humanity's cooperative nature.

Doctors and patients, teachers and pupils, writers and readers, bees and flowers, even viruses and hosts, are in this dance together. We're connected by invisible threads too remote to measure. Our connections remain much stronger, much more solid than the distance and the deceptions and the hatred that divides.

Maybe I figured this wrong, searching for threads here and there. A million threads link us to our shared humanity. So much connects us — love, history, the web of causality, the air we all breathe, the water we drink, even our common grief. Our sorrows and chains and plight hold choices and possibilities.

I loitered on the bench on my hill. I belonged here. Yeah, it's my hill. Here I loaf, so here I must belong. And here I arrange space for you, dear reader, to also linger with these reflections. Off to the left towered the steel and glass of downtown. To the right, in the west, stood the endless winter white line of the Rockies. Our neighbourhood lay beneath my feet, the roofs glazed with a snow frosting. Grey and white smoke rose from each house's chimney, like an idyllic fairy tale village.

At this crucial moment in history, I can choose kindness over resentments, action over despair. In some tiny, inconsequential way, I can help pull the world back from crazy. Let loose the Buddha from my belly. Happy or sad, today, I am alive.

On the bench I knew: life has blessed me in every way. The little boy whose stomach hurt won. And now, unprepared, but willingly, I face our common tumultuous future. So bring on the madness and the beauty. Let's raise a glass; sing cheers to this new beginning. Let me inhale, taste, digest it all.

Under the tree, the Buddha vowed to save all living beings. Back then, he didn't know that beings live inside us. Our guts provide homes to some thirty trillion invisible bacteria, viruses, protists, archaea, and fungi. Them tiny critters need love too. Allow our truest selves to issue forth from the deep, tender, resilient centre. Sing the songs of our wild, precious selves in our unique words, to our chosen beat. Others will hear and sing in return.

My eyes closed. I tilted my face up to the afternoon sun and slight chill in the air. My neck relaxed and shoulders solidly pulled back. Not overwhelmed, just nicely whelmed. Everything due to my parents and brothers, my mentor and partner, countless others, Earth herself, the life-force itself. To pay them back, I'll keep looking for the words. Give voice to the Buddha in my belly.

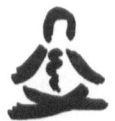

# The question of the bench

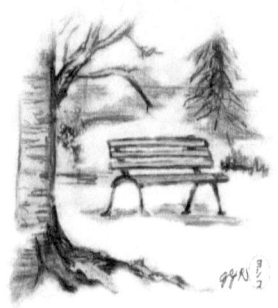

In the city park just
around the corner,
at the end of a twisted
trail.
on a boardwalk by the
beach,
the bench waits.

At night the gates locked,
All day as hikers pass,
After we've flown home,
the bench waits.

Whatever long meandering steps
brought you,
Hesitant, purposeful or noncha-
lant,
Graceful, trudging or malevolent
— You arrive.
The bench has waited.

# THE QUESTION OF THE BENCH

Have a sit.
Shake the pebble from your shoe,
See the mountain within reach.
Don't feed the squirrels or ducks.
Smell the sea.


A moment alone,
Lover in your arms,
Grandchild on your lap,
Puppy's eyes look up.


Enjoy this moment, this day.
Sun against your cheek.
Rain on your hood.
Sandwich, falafel or rice ball


Have a sit and think about your life.
What do you want?
What are you doing with your life?
The bench no longer waits.
The wait is over.
What are you doing with your life?

# EPILOGUE

After eleven major surgeries, myriad procedures, and hospitalizations, here I rise. May these stories encourage seeing possibilities where now might be despair. A long time ago, I fled an LA welfare office filled with shame, regret, and self loathing. Every opportunity wasted, I thought. Out of options. Fortunately, I could not have been more wrong. My story had barely begun.

Here we are, dear reader, at the epilogue, the end. More than a medical memoir, my story is about identity and belonging — where do I fit? Maybe identity is neither inborn nor discovered. Perhaps we create identity through our choices, our thoughts, words, and deeds. Once created, we nurture who we are, elevate this thing we call a self as we raise a child or a fine wine sleeping in a cave. Then we adapt to a changing world and the creation commences again.

Being afflicted with Crohn's is my reality. With this disease, I found purpose. My experience with Crohn's is a role, but not who I am. My story became about options, about making choices and creating choices where none seem to exist.

We are like actors performing roles, my mentor taught: "You are the playwright of your own victory. You are also the play's hero ... Neither chance nor a divine being writes the script for us. We write it, and we are the actors who play it."[64]

As I write this, Daisaku and Kaneko are both healthy, although no longer travelling. He turned ninety-four in 2022, and she is ninety-two. They both still encourage others daily, writing and working for peace and for the human revolution. The week I spent with them in Sceaux defined my life, but nothing like I imagined. Life is so much richer, wondrous, and so much more colourful and beautiful than my black and white imagination.

# EPILOGUE

Recently I went to a dedicated clinic for my regular six-week infliximab infusion. Along with her forget-me-not eyes, I inherited Mom's thin, rolling veins with lots of valves. Nurses proclaim my veins "a hard start." For two hours, I laze on an overstuffed, reclining La-Z-Boy chair. Four or five other immune-compromised folks also receive infusions. We enjoy choices of juices and Peek Freans cookies while the biologic TNF blockers pump into our veins. Between offering us treats, the nurses check our vitals and pose questions about our health since our last infusions.

On this occasion, a friend of Andrea's, who also has CD, fundraised for the Crohn's and Colitis Society. She requested I wear a T-shirt to this infusion. The shirt had the slogan, "I hate my guts" across the front. Clever. And take a picture for social media. You bet, delighted to.

What a delight to join these bright young campaigners, even virtually. They refuse to be victims; our disease does not define them. Some are gravely ill, a few with ostomies. Not merely soliciting donations, they champion all those with inflammatory bowel disease. They rise for those who cannot stand, suffering in lonely privies and bedrooms and hospital wards.

Crohn's will not defeat these courageous young people. Their vision goes beyond their own suffering to how they can contribute. The campaign used pictures of them and a lone beaming balding fat old guy.

I wore the T-shirt but didn't accept the slogan. No longer do I hate my guts. Although I only enjoy a few remaining feet, I love and appreciate my intestines. They have nourished and cared for me through it all. Despite rejection, they deliver nutrients and keep out toxins, creating the soil for me to blossom.

The Crohn's remains in remission. My intestines are now perfect — soft and baby pink, hale and hearty. During my kidney issue, I had a colonoscopy. More recently I went for a screening CT colonography (sometimes called a virtual colonoscopy.) My guts are like me — soft and pink and happy.

Inside and out, I am realizing peace.

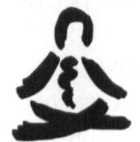

# MY GLOSSARY

As mentioned in the INTRODUCTION, the following are my explanations of Buddhist terms I use. The explanations are not those you will find in a book or class on Buddhism. They are entirely my own understanding and intended to be helpful in the context of this book. For explanations of medical terminology used in the text, and for further exploration of Crohn's disease, hidradenitis suppurativa, and Nichiren Buddhism, see the RESOURCES section at the end.

## Bodhisattva

A person who works to relieve the suffering of others. The personification of compassionate behaviour.

## Dharma

Dharma means three related things: the teachings of the Buddha (the Law), the phenomena the teachings apply to, and the conduct implied by the teaching. For example, one teaching of Buddhism is causality, what the Buddha called "contingent arising" or "dependent origination." All things everywhere, throughout time, exist in relation to all other things. Nothing exists without a cause for its existence. Everything is connected and interdependent. In this example, dharma refers to both the principle of causality and the things (all phenomena) the principle applies to.

Using the same example of contingent arising, nothing is fully independent. Therefore, behaviour in the world as if one is independent is foolish and will lead to poor effects (on others, if not oneself). Behaviour mindful of our interdependence is wise and will lead to positive effects.

This third meaning is not tertiary or derivative. I believe the Buddha's primary intention was not to define a new set of dogmas, but to improve human behaviour. The Buddha's teachings are neither dogma nor absolutes, to be believed or not, accepted or not. They are calls to ethical action.

## Lotus Sutra

The sutras are the teachings attributed to the Buddha. The word "sutra" originally meant string of cloth. Our modern words "suture" (surgical thread), "couture" (dress making, fashion), "souvlaki" (skewered meat) all derive from the same proto-Indo-European root.

Long after the Buddha's death around 400 BCE, the first written records of his teachings began to be compiled. These were what we now call the sutras. Many dozens of sutras exist today. None of them date back anywhere near the Buddha's lifetime. They wildly contradict each other, are internally inconsistent, and often contain obvious embellishments.

Even today's scholars, historians, and philologists peer under the contradictions and embellishments to find patterns and an evolution of Buddhist thinking. Between the first century BCE and third century CE, that evolution reached its apex with the compilation of the Lotus Sutra (Sanskrit: Saddharma Puṇḍarīka Sūtra). The Lotus attempts to unite the varying doctrines while returning to the Buddha's original intention of saving all beings.

The Lotus Sutra teaches that every person has the inner potential to experience wisdom, compassion, and life force. That potential is both inherent to life itself and co-existent with the great cosmos. Nothing can take away that energy for transformation; it is eternal and immanent to all beings and the environment.

"Known as the 'King of Sutras, the Lotus Sutra is one of the most influential texts in East Asian Buddhism,"[65] and is regarded "as a religious classic of great beauty and power."[66]

If the scriptures of Abrahamic religions—the Torah, Bible, Quran—are considered Revealed Truth (capitals intentional), the sutras can be considered as revealing of truths. Rather than historical fact, the sutras express the grandeur and wonder of each life within the cosmic web.

## Nichiren (literally, Sun-Lotus)

1222–1283 Japanese priest and founder of the Buddhist tradition I practise. Nichiren's teachings are based on the Lotus Sutra, the conviction in the inherent dignity of all beings. He believed everyone can experience the Buddha's awakening, not just clergy or professionals. He believed that every person of any gender, rich or poor, foolish or wise, saint or sinner, has the potential for a caring, full life. Enlightenment, he thought, was humanity's destiny.

Nichiren spent twenty years studying the entirety of the canon available — sutras, commentaries, and doctrines of the various schools. He concluded that the purpose of Buddhism was to elevate all people to their highest potentialities and to build a peaceful land. He distilled the teachings into an accessible practice — recitation of the formula Nam-myoho-renge-kyo. Myoho-renge-kyo is the title, Wondrous Dharma of the Lotus Sutra, and Nam is an expression of praise or devotion.

Nichiren aimed to return Buddhism to its original purpose of guiding people to their awakening, while establishing a practice "that would supersede existing forms."[67] He severely criticized the established Buddhist schools of his time. He rejected their cleric centred elitism and alliances with political authority. He rejected their teaching that enlightenment was not available to women nor to commoners, that relief from suffering existed only after death. Their temples and livelihood depended on official government support. As a result, Nichiren experienced a lifetime of persecution and hardships. He was physically attacked, exiled twice, and the authorities attempted to execute him. His followers were also persecuted — some were imprisoned or executed, their lands confiscated.

# ACKNOWLEDGEMENTS

*The Buddha in Our Bellies* would not be possible without the contributions of many. In particular, we are deeply indebted to (in no order):

Prema Naidu and Saroja Subramanian Iyer, for their meticulous assistance in conceiving Yasodhara's sari.

*New Century* "August 2018," SGI Canada's monthly magazine, for previously publishing portions of "My Quest."

Justine Evans, RN (Retired), Bachelor of Health Science (Nursing), for medical review, peer review, and wise encouragement.

Nidhi Bhatia, for patient and thoughtful sensitivity review.

Annie and Aurore Bourla, for reviewing the chapter "Friday the 13th," and for their persistent friendship and constant encouragement. *Gros bisous, Mesdames.*

Yusaku Yamamoto, for family research. *Oniichan, arigatou gozaimashita.*

Erica, for choosing us. Andrea, for carrying us over the finish line.

Esther Castain, our editor.

# ACKNOWLEDGEMENTS

Traci Skuce, for mentoring and coaching. If you are interested in improving your writing and telling your stories, chat with Traci, https://www.traciskuce.com/>. Thank you, Traci, for teaching me where to put the bodies.

Christina Poniecki, MA in Psychology, C.H.T., for feedback and encouragement, for Sicamous squashes that fed us through the cold writing winters, for Hakomi Therapy to keep me centred and in my body.

All pre-publication readers. Your contribution has been mighty.

Myron Hyrak, for layout, design, and for believing we had Buddhas in our bellies.

Calgary Gosho Study Group, for encouragement and weekly study of Nichiren's writings.

Arianna Occhipinti, for her wisdom, permission to tell our story of meeting, and her extraordinary wines. *Grazij. Gracie mille.* From across the continents and waters, we bow to you.

Janet Surrey and Samuel Shem, authors of *The Buddha's Wife: The Path of Awakening Together*, Atria Books, 2015 for planting the seed of Yasodhara's enlightenment in our mind. Depictions of Yasodhara's character, dialogue, and actions, however, are wholly our own.

Dr. Swarna Prabha, Ph.D, Associate Professor of Hindi (ret.), Delhi University, Daulat Ram College, for assistance with depicting Indian life in the fifth century BCE. Any errors or omissions are our own.

Sunaina Sindhwani, author of *The Purple Couch*, and Prashant Publications for assistance with the India edition.

# RESOURCES

For information on Crohn's disease:
Canada  crohnsandcolitis.ca
U.S.A.  crohnscolitisfoundation.org
U.K.  crohnsandcolitis.org.uk
E.U.  efcca.org

For information on Soka Gakkai:
Global  sokaglobal.org/resources/related-websites.html
Canada  sgicanada.org
India  bharatsokagakkai.org
USA  sgi-usa.org
UK  sgi-uk.org
France  soka-bouddhisme.fr

For information on hidradenitis suppurativa (HS):
Canada  hsfoundation.ca/en
USA  aad.org/public/diseases/a-z/hidradenitis-suppurativa-treatment
Europe  hs-institute.com

To reach the authors of *The Buddha in Our Bellies*:
pilgrimsofjoy@gmail.com

1. "Fatigue and autoimmune disease,"
   Harvard Medical School, Harvard Health Publishing,
   (October 14, 2022),
   <https://www.health.harvard.edu/diseases-and-conditions/fatigue-and-autoimmune-disease>

2. Megan O'Rourke, "What's Wrong with Me?"
   The New Yorker (August 26, 2013)
   <https://www.newyorker.com/magazine/2013/08/26/whats-wrong-with-me/>

3. Mark Musa, trans., Dante's Vita Nuova
   (Bloomington: Indiana UP, 1973),
   p 3

4. Jordan E. Rosenfeld, "The WD Interview: Isabel Allende,"
   Writer's Digest, (August 27, 2008)
   <https://www.writersdigest.com/memoir-by-writing-genre/isabel-allende>

5. Daisaku Ikeda,
   "Quotations by theme — Human Revolution,"
   <https://www.daisakuikeda.org/sub/quotations/theme/human-revolution.html>

6. Donald S. Lopez, Jr., "The Life of the Lotus Sutra," Tricycle Magazine (Winter 2016),
   <https://tricycle.org/magazine/lotus-sutra-history/>

7. Burton Watson, trans., The Lotus Sutra and Its Opening and Closing Sutras (LSOC),
   (Tokyo: Soka Gakkai, 1999), p 159

8. George Dunea, "Fabricius Hildanus – father of German surgery,"
   Hektoen International Journal 7, 2 (Spring 2015),
   <https://hekint.org/2017/01/22/fabricius-hildanus-father-of-german-surgery/>

9. R. Nagle, "'A Singular Case' and Dr. Smethurst," Medico-Legal Journal 38, 2 (June 1970):51,
   <https://doi.org/10.1177/002581727003800203>

10. Dara Mohammadi, "The curious case of inflammatory bowel disease," The Lancet 1, 2 (October 2016): 94,
    <https://doi.org/10.1016/S2468-1253(16)30091-7>

11. "Trial Of Thomas Smethurst," The British Medical Journal (August 27, 1859): 709–10,
    <https://www.google.com/books/edition/British_Medical_Journal/dvtGAQAAMAAJ?hl=en&gbpv=0>

12. A. Newton, The Case of Thomas Smethurst, MD (London: Routledge, Warne, & Rotledge, 1859), pp87–90,
    <https://iiif.lib.harvard.edu/manifests/view/drs:5787363$8i>

13. Dara Mohammadi, "The curious case of inflammatory bowel disease," The Lancet 1, 2 (October 2016): 94,
    <https://doi.org/10.1016/S2468-1253(16)30091-7>

14. Burrill B. Crohn , L Ginzburg, G.D. Oppenheimer, "Regional Ileitis: A Pathologic And Clinical Entity," Journal of the American Medical Association. 1932;99(16):1323–1329.
    <https://jamanetwork.com/journals/jama/article-abstract/286298>

15. Fábio Guilherme M. C. Campos and Paulo Gustavo Kotze, "Burrill Bernard Crohn (1884–1983): o homem por trás da doença (the man behind the disease)," ABCD. Arquivos Brasileiros de Cirurgia Digestiva (São Paulo), 2013 26(4), 253–255.
    <https://doi.org/10.1590/S0102-67202013000400001>

16. Joseph B. Kirsner, "Historical origins of current IBD concepts," World Journal of Gastroenterology 7, no. 2 (April 2001):178,
    <https://doi.org/10.3748/wjg.v7.i2.175>

17. Joshua R. Korzenik, "Past and Current Theories of Etiology of IBD: Toothpaste, Worms, and Refrigerators," Journal of Clinical Gastroenterology 39, 4 (April 2005): S59–S65, <https://doi.org/10.1097/01.mcg.0000155553.28348.fc>

18. Crohn's and Colitis Canada, 2018 Impact of Inflammatory Bowel Disease in Canada, p 12, <https://crohnsandcolitis.ca/Crohns_and_Colitis/documents/reports/2018-Impact-Report-LR.pdf>

19. James M. Dahlhamer, Emily P. Zammitti, et al., "Prevalence of Inflammatory Bowel Disease Among Adults Aged ≥18 Years — United States, 2015," Morbidity and Mortality Weekly Report, no. 42 (October 28, 2016):1166, <http://dx.doi.org/10.15585/mmwr.mm6542a3>

20. Katherine Chang, "What It's Like Living with Crohn's," The Everygirl blog (November 10, 2018), <https://theeverygirl.com/what-its-like-living-with-crohns/>

21. "First Signs of My IBD," 'Experience Journal', compiled by Boston Children's Hospital, <https://experiencejournal.com/journals/inflammatory-bowel-disease-ibd/first-signs-of-my-ibd/>

22. Quoted in Jennifer Dobson, "Invisible Illness and Measurability," AMA Journal of Ethics 23, no. 7 (July 2021):E512, <https://doi.org/10.1001/amajethics.2021.402>

23. Interview by Paul Costello, "My rendezvous with insanity," Stanford Medicine (Fall 2014), <https://stanmed.stanford.edu/my-rendezvous-with-insanity/>

24. Rebecca C Spillmann, Allyn McConkie-Rosell, et al., "A window into living with an undiagnosed disease: illness narratives from the Undiagnosed Diseases Network," Orphanet Journal of Rare Diseases 12, 71 (2017), pp 1, 2, 4, <https://doi.org/10.1186/s13023-017-0623-3>

25. Daisaku Ikeda, Katsuji Saito, et al.,
    The Wisdom of the Lotus Sutra (WLS), Volume IV
    (Santa Monica: World Tribune Press, 2002) pp 120, 122

26. Nichiren, WND, Volume II, p 197

27. Originally published in 1921 by Ujō Noguchi as "Karesusuki"
    [Withered Pampas].
    Lyrics translated by Yoshiko and Keith Robinson

28. "Internment in Siberia: Background to the Internment of Japanese People in the USSR,"
    Maizuru Repatriation Memorial Museum website,
    <https://m-hikiage-museum.jp/english-education/03-ussr.html>.
    The Soviets captured and held around six hundred thousand Japanese civilians and military personnel.

29. "Gulag," History website, last updated January 11, 2023
    (A&E Television Networks),
    <https://www.history.com/topics/european-history/gulag>

30. English lyrics translation of "Akatonbo" [Red Dragonfly]
    by Norio Shimizu,
    <https://lyricstranslate.com/en/red-dragonflies-lyrics.html>.
    Used with permission

31. "1968: East Los Angeles Walkouts," A Latinx Resource Guide:
    Civil Rights Cases and Events in the United States,
    Library of Congress Research Guides
    <https://guides.loc.gov/latin"-civil-rights/east-la-walkouts>

32. Daisaku Ikeda, The New Human Revolution (NHR), Volume 14
    (Santa Monica: World Tribune Press, 2007), p 4

33. Ibid., p 10

34. Megan O'Rourke, "What's Wrong with Me?"
    The New Yorker (August 26, 2013)
    <https://www.newyorker.com/magazine/2013/08/26/whats-wrong-with-me/>

35. Ibid.

36. Jennifer Dobson, "Invisible Illness and Measurability," AMA Journal of Ethics 23, no. 7 (July 2021): E512, <https://doi.org/10.1001/amajethics.2021.402>

37. Ibid.

38. Daisaku Ikeda, "Ode to Youth," in Lectures on the Gosho (Tokyo: Soka University English Academy, 1976), p 145

39. Daisaku Ikeda, "Chapter 8.3: Chanting Nam-myoho-renge-kyo Is the Wellspring of Life Force," The Wisdom for Creating Happiness and Peace series (WCHP), Part 1 <https://www.sokaglobal.org/resources/study-materials/buddhist-study/the-wisdom-for-creating-happiness-and-peace/chapter-8-3.html>

40. Richard Hofstadter, American Political Tradition and the Men Who Made It (New York: Alfred Knopf 1948), x.

41. Daisaku Ikeda, "Chapter 1.5: Creating a Life of Genuine Freedom," WCHP, Part 1 <https://www.sokaglobal.org/resources/study-materials/buddhist-study/the-wisdom-for-creating-happiness-and-peace/chapter-1-5.html>

42. James Baldwin, Notes of a Native Son (Boston: Beacon Press, 1984), p 123

43. Carlos Ruiz Zafón, The Shadow of the Wind, trans. by Lucia Graves (London: Penguin Books, 2001), p 68

44. Travels for Peace (Tokyo: Seikyo Shimbun, 1972), p 65

45. John Ciardi, trans.,
    Dante Alighieri, Inferno,
    (New York: The Modern Library, 1996),
    p 3

46. Ira M. Robinson, An Urban Life Journey from the Bronx, NYC to Victoria, BC (Winnipeg: Gemma Publishing, 2011), p 85

47. Martin Luther King, Jr., Strength To Love, (New York: A Pocket Book, 1963), p 88

48. Nichiren, WND Volume I, p 166

49. Jimmy Akin, "Excommunication: It's Not What You Think," Catholic Answers (October 25, 2021) <https://www.catholic.com/magazine/online-edition/excommunication-its-not-what-you-think>

50. James Baldwin, The Fire Next Time (New York: The Modern Library, 1995), p 8

51. Burton Watson, trans, LSOC, chapter 6, p 146

52. In India it's in September and is called Pitra Paksha - days of gone ancestors. In China it is called the Yulanpen Festival In Indonesia, Sembahyang Cioko. In Japan, The Bon Festival. In Vietnam, Tết Trung Nguyên. Laos, Boun khao padap din. Thailand, Sat Thai. Customs vary from country to country, but all share similar roots of respect for the deceased and some form of hungry spirits being released from the prison of craving.

53. Vivian Gornick, "Memory Palace,"
    Los Angeles Times (September 26, 1992), <https://www.latimes.com/archives/la-xpm-1999-sep-26-bk-14162-story.html>

54. Siri Carpenter, "That gut feeling," Monitor on Psychology 43, no 8 (September 2012),
    <http://www.apa.org/monitor/2012/09/gut-feeling>

55. Premysl Bercik, Emmanuel Denou, et al., "The intestinal microbiota affect central levels of brain-derived neurotropic factor and behavior in mice," Gastroenterology 141(2) (August 2011): P599-609, 609.e1-3,
<https://doi.org/10.1053/j.gastro.2011.04.052>

56. See Tanya T Nguyen, Xinliang Zhang, et al., "Association of Loneliness and Wisdom With Gut Microbial Diversity and Composition: An Exploratory Study," Frontiers in Psychiatry 12 (March 25, 2021), <https://doi.org/10.3389/fpsyt.2021.648475>

57. Charles Hallisey, trans.,
Poems of the First Buddhist Women, A Translation of the Therigatha (Cambridge: Harvard UP, 2021), p 51

58. Matty Weingast, The First Free Women: Poems of the Early Buddhist Nuns
(Boulder: Shambhala Publications, 2020),
p 93

59. John Ciardi, trans., Dante Alighieri, Inferno, (New York: The Modern Library, 1996), p 309

60. WHO, "Coronavirus (COVID-19) Dashboard" <https://covid19.who.int/>

61. See LSOC chapter 8, pp 190–191

62. Burton Watson, trans. The Record of the Orally Transmitted Teachings [by Nichiren] (Tokyo: Soka Gakkai, 2004), p 211

63. Nichiren, WND, Volume I, p 536

64. Qtd in SGI-USA "Encouragement" blog, (November 1, 2014), <https://web.archive.org/web/20180329172031/https://www.sgi-usa.org/2014/11/01/you-are-the-playwright-of-your-own-victory/>

65. James Shaheen, Tricycle Magazine (Spring 2020), <https://tricycle.org/magazine/how-to-read-the-lotus-sutra/>

66. Britannica, The Editors of Encyclopaedia. "Lotus Sutra," Encyclopedia Britannica, 20 May. 2013, <https://www.britannica.com/topic/Lotus-Sutra>

67. Jacqueline Stone, "Knowing Nichiren," Tricycle Magazine, (Spring 2023) <https://tricycle.org/magazine/nichiren-buddhism-history/>

www.ingramcontent.com/pod-product-compliance
Lightning Source LLC
Chambersburg PA
CBHW032358100526
44587CB00010BA/221